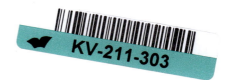

Interprofessional Education:
An agenda for healthcare professionals

edited by
Caroline Carlisle, Tom Donovan and Dave Mercer

With a foreword by Sir Kenneth Calman

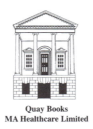

Quay Books
MA Healthcare Limited

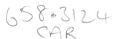

Quay Books Division, MA Healthcare Limited, Jesses Farm, Snow Hill, Dinton, Salisbury, Wiltshire, SP3 5HN

British Library Cataloguing-in-Publication Data
A catalogue record is available for this book

© MA Healthcare Limited 2005
ISBN 1 85642 238 0

Printed in the UK by Cromwell Press Limited, Trowbridge, Wiltshire

Contents

About the contributors

Hugh Barr is Chair of the UK Centre for the Advancement of Interprofessional Education (IPE) and has many years' experience in the field of IPE. He is Emeritus Professor of IPE at the University of Westminster and Editor-in-Chief of the *Journal of Interprofessional Care*. He has written extensively on the subject of IPE and his publications include key works for the Learning and Teaching Support Network. He has particular interest and experience in the evaluation of IPE.

Phil Blundell is senior lecturer in mental health nursing at the University of Central Lancashire. Much of his work focuses on how teams operate within a multiprofessional framework, and he has worked closely with a number of teams within their own clinical environments. Recently he was a major developer of the National Demonstration Project, a programme designed to deliver training to all members of healthcare teams at ten pilot sites. As a key facilitator in this project, he enabled teams to review and change their working practices and to explore the dynamics within their own teams.

Lyn Brown worked for the Child Care Service and Probation Service in the 1960s, and spent four years with the Prison Probation Department in a male prison before becoming a teacher in social work and medical education at the University of Liverpool. She is currently responsible for the 'Caring in the Community' course, a programme that places medical students with agencies concerned in health and social care. Students are encouraged to understand the community through 'the patient's eyes' and explore the roles of local organisations that offer support. Lyn has also researched and written on support for families bereaved through multiple homicide and victim support for the families of murder victims.

Caroline Carlisle has a professional background in primary care having worked for many years as a district nurse, practice nurse and community midwife. She is currently Professor of Education in Nursing and Midwifery at the University of Manchester. She teaches a range of subjects to healthcare professionals, including communication and consultation skills, and research design. Her research field is the area of women's health and sexual health,and she has a specific interest in education for advanced practice roles for nurses.

Kate Cernik is an experienced nurse, health visitor and educator. As lead nurse at a PMS practice in Appleton, Warrington, she is developing interprofessional approaches to the delivery of primary care services, and has been involved in developing nursing practice, particularly around nurse prescribing. Kate is also an education adviser with the University of Liverpool Postgraduate General Practice Office. Her main area of work has been to foster interprofessional approaches to educational activities for GPs, other clinicians and support staff in primary care. In addition, she manages a portfolio of communication skills courses for practitioners and others working in primary care.

Helen Cooper has a professional background in diabetes nursing and health visiting. Her research is centred on patient education and undergraduate IPE. She has acted as an expert adviser and provided evidence to inform the National Institute for Clinical Excellence report on patient education models for diabetes. She was involved in reviewing diabetes professional education for the Medical Research Council. She is currently a lecturer in healthcare education and Coordinator for IPE at the University of Liverpool.

Tom Donovan is a Macmillan lecturer in the Department of Nursing at the University of Liverpool, where he is currently Adult Branch Leader for the pre-registration undergraduate programme. His recent experience encompasses roles in cancer and palliative care settings. He has worked as a clinical nurse specialist and was lead cancer nurse to the Royal Liverpool University Hospital until 2002. His research interests include the psychosocial care of people with cancer and communication skills training. He is presently undertaking PhD studies, and is also researching the experiences of patients undergoing rapid diagnosis for cancer.

Mike Farrell qualified as a registered general nurse in 1984 and further trained as a children's nurse. He has gained most of his experience in the care of the critically ill child, having had several positions in general and specialist paediatric intensive care settings. In 1994 he was appointed senior nurse at Derian House Children's Hospice, and from 1998 until 2003 he worked as a lecturer/practitioner in the Department of Nursing, University of Liverpool, and the Royal Liverpool Children's NHS Trust. He is currently Project Manager at the Cumbria and Lancashire Workforce Development Confederation, with responsibility for the development of an e-learning strategy.

Sally Gosling is Head of Learning and Development at the Chartered Society of Physiotherapy. She coordinates strategic work on qualifying and post-qualifying physiotherapy education, and leads on a range of activities relating to regulatory change. She is currently managing a Department of Health-funded project across the allied health professions on demonstrating competence through continuing professional development. Sally sits on a number of interprofessional groups concerned with healthcare education, including those convened by the Quality Assurance Agency and the Advisory Board for the Learning and Teaching Support Network for Health Sciences and Practice.

Caroline Haigh is a trainee clinical psychologist at the University of Surrey, Guildford. At the time of the work discussed in this book, she was a research assistant attached to the University of Central Lancashire.

Marilyn Hammick's research interests include education systematic reviews, cancer fatigue and research supervision. Work on an evidence base for IPE has involved her in developing effective ways of measuring educational outcomes. Marilyn is Vice-chair of the Centre for the Advancement of Interprofessional Education, Associate Editor of the *Journal of Interprofessional Care,* and is on the steering committee of the Best Evidence Medical Education Group. Her previous posts were at the Centre for Research in Medical & Dental Education, University of Birmingham, Director of Quality and Head of Department of Professional Studies, Oxford Brookes University, and in clinical cancer care.

Anne Lanceley is a Clinical Nursing Research Fellow in gynaecological cancer at Queen Mary's School of Medicine and Dentistry, London. Anne has been caring for cancer patients since 1981 and has held several innovative clinical posts, including nurse lead to the first teenage cancer unit in Europe. Anne has a lifelong interest in language and communication, and read English literature at London University before her doctoral research. This looked at the processes and emotional content of talk between nurses and cancer patients and examined the impact on the nurses of hearing patients' distress. Her current research themes are communication and interprofessional working.

Julie Lord is senior nurse for the service development team at Wigan Borough Partnership NHS Trust. Julie is currently on secondment to the Sainsbury Centre for Mental Health, London, where she is project manager for the Acute In-patient Diploma course.

Di Marks-Maran is a consultant in healthcare education, and formerly Professor of Nursing Education at Thames Valley University. She is currently undertaking independent consultancy to a number of healthcare faculties in universities across the UK. Before this she was Head of the Centre for Teaching and Learning. In that role she led the development of distance- and problem-based learning in the faculty, using social constructivist theory as the basis for these initiatives. Her main areas of interest are enabling academic staff to develop their potential for scholarship in practice, open and distance learning, e-learning, and social constructivism and its application in practice.

Mick McKeown is principal lecturer in mental health nursing research at the University of Central Lancashire. He has a longstanding interest in issues of service-user involvement, especially in inpatient settings, and is a trade union activist for Unison and a member of the Government's Standing Nursing and Midwifery Advisory Committee. Mick has published widely, including scholarly papers on psychosocial interventions in secure care, the social construction of race and mental health, professional understandings of risk, drug use and psychosis. He has jointly edited a new book *Forensic Mental Health Care: A Case Study Approach*, published by Churchill Livingstone.

Dave Mercer is a lecturer in the Department of Nursing at the University of Liverpool. His first degree and postgraduate studies were in sociology and criminology, respectively. Critical social theory has informed and guided his career as a mental health nurse in terms of practice, research and education. He has a wide range of publications on the care and management of the mentally disordered offender, many of which explore professional discourses in terms of institutionalised power and ideology. Dave has a particular interest in teaching communication and interpersonal skills as a fundamental ingredient of healthcare practice, and encouraging students to engage with the personal, professional and political dimensions of language.

Tim Riding qualified as a registered nurse for the mentally handicapped in 1988, initially working within the high security learning disability services. He then joined a community learning disability team, first as senior clinical specialist in challenging behaviour and latterly as a nurse consultant. In this role, in addition to carrying a caseload of people with complex needs, Tim was also responsible for developing clinical practice and contributing to the development of an evidence base for learning disability nursing. Tim has recently taken up the post of Secure Services Network Director at Lancashire Care NHS Trust.

Ray Sutton is the founder and manager of Actor/Educators Inc, a company specialising in healthcare communication skills training. He performs regularly with the company as a simulated patient or relative. He was formerly Head of Drama at Liverpool's John Moores University. He has published on communication skills in drama, clinician in management and medical education.

Philip Turner trained as a speech and language therapist, qualifying in 1978. He held a series of clinical posts before becoming the service manager in Tameside and Glossop. He has fulfilled a range of duties for his professional body, the Royal College of Speech and Language Therapists. In 1993 he moved to Chester and Halton to become the manager of a range of therapy services. In 2000 he was seconded to the NHS Executive (Northwest) to undertake a project developing networks for the allied health professions. He currently fulfils a number of service management and strategic roles for Halton primary care trust.

Gill Young is a Reader in Educational Development at Thames Valley University. She is currently project managing evaluation research into the Faculty of Health and Human Science's learning communities development. She carried out evaluation research on the two projects described in the case studies in *Chapter 12*. Currently, her main areas of interest are the development of research and scholarship, open and distance learning and e-learning, social constructivism, learning organisations and IPE.

Foreword

The term 'interprofessional education' (IPE) is an interesting one. It has three components, the first of which relates to the broad concept of a profession and the values and boundaries that each professional group sets up around it. The second is education and the process of learning. The third is the 'inter' which brings together these two concepts across professional divisions.

Professions do have several things in common. They all have a particular knowledge base, they all have special links between the client/patient and the professional, and they all have values that are of great importance to them. They generally have the privilege of being able to set their own examinations, and thus their own standards. In most instances they are self-regulating. Education, of course, is also about values and the ways in which each profession ensures that those who are part of it meet the criteria of entry and continuing accreditation.

Putting all of these components together for each professional group, with the associated boundaries, inevitably leads to tension. How can the knowledge base of a speech therapist be the same as that of a pharmacist? How do the values of a social worker and a nurse relate to each other? How can the educational processes to gain entry to each profession be the same? How can continuing professional development be similar for each group? The learning processes, of course, are the same, as are the methods and the assessments, but the end-point, as expressed in terms of knowledge, skills and attitudes, may be quite different. What then is the rationale for IPE and why is it so important?

The basic outcome of the learning of any individual from any of the many professions involved in health and social care is to be able to care effectively for the patient or client for whom he or she has a particular responsibility. As the range of knowledge and skills has expanded, so new professional groups have developed to meet the needs of individual patients. It becomes clear that no single professional group can cover all the ground and provide all that is required for each patient, hence the need to work in teams and to share experience and skills across the professions.

IPE therefore has two aims. The first is to recognise the boundaries and limitations of each individual and professional group. The second is to learn about the skills and experience of others. In one sense, the learning processes, for example, lectures, group work and problem-solving sessions, are secondary to our own limitations and our ability to recognise the skills of others and work effectively alongside them as members of a team. With the increasing complexity of health and social care, such issues are likely to become more pressing, hence the need to begin to tackle the problems now. As the environment within which patient care is delivered also changes, so the individual professional will have to deal with an increasing and varied workload, and will find her or his colleagues in different professions doing the same. The development of organisational models, such as managed care packages, and the huge expansion of new knowledge, and even new subjects, make the issue of pressing importance. The sooner we can get to grips with the problems the better it will be for our patients. At the heart of the process are the wish and the willingness to do the best for the patient/client.

How can this best be done? It has already been acknowledged that the range of learning methods is considerable and that these should facilitate the process, the method being chosen to fit the learning objectives. This aspect of IPE should not be an issue. The bigger problem is to set the learning objectives themselves. What do we really want to achieve within the broad aims set out above? This is the most difficult part of the process and may take time to develop. First, there needs to be an agreement that patients and the public are part of the process and an important learning resource. The expertise of those who have been affected by illness is considerable, and patients should be seen as an integral part of the team. Second, each professional group must learn to respect each other and to recognise each other's skills. One objective would be to identify the roles and expertise of each profession. This can be readily achieved through joint problem-solving exercises, during which the real role of each profession becomes clearer. In primary care, the development of practice development plans and audits of specific processes and outcomes can identify new areas for learning.

In all of this, we need evidence of effectiveness at the level of patient care. More evidence is needed, together with innovative ways of enhancing the learning. Such evidence is beginning to emerge, and some of it is set out in this book. The more we can share such information the better. Fortunately, there are now a number of organisations that provide a forum for such debates. The Association for the Study of Medical Education (ASME) and the UK Centre for the Advancement of Interprofessional Education (CAIPE) are two such groups. The literature needs to be expanded and developed, and all professions need to show willingness to discuss and debate the concerns and excitement of working together. Our patients deserve it, and that is what matters.

Kenneth C Calman
Durham 2004

Introduction

The past decade has seen increasing interest in, and activity related to, interprofessional education (IPE). Papers on the topic feature regularly in professional healthcare and education journals, and organisations such as the Centre for the Advancement of Interprofessional Education (CAIPE) do much to promote debate and scholarly activity in the field. IPE is explicitly featured in current educational and healthcare policy agenda (Department of Health, 2000). Many higher education institutions are developing educational strategies that acknowledge the importance of IPE across faculties, not solely in health care. There is no doubt that faculties of health care need to find ways to effectively implement IPE across traditional professional boundaries, which enable all professionals to see the relevance of the content to their own clinical practice.

In structuring this present volume, we set out to provide a straightforward and topical critique of IPE from the perspective of a range of healthcare professionals, and to present some useful examples of the ways in which IPE is implemented in both educational and clinical settings. The contributors to this text come from a variety of health profession backgrounds: some work mainly in clinical practice, while others have their primary responsibility in management or education.

The book is presented in two parts. **Part 1 (Interprofessional education in context)** aims to provide a detailed account of the IPE agenda, including a review of the current contextual climate, the agenda relating to healthcare education, and the debate on the potential value of the IPE approach. Developing a shared definition of IPE is essential if healthcare educators and providers are to take a strategic approach to effectively implementing IPE. The book therefore begins by debating terminology and exploring the current presence, or absence, of the evidence base for IPE (*Chapter 1*).

In *Chapter 2*, Sally Gosling, a physiotherapist, explores the drivers for, as well as the barriers to, the implementation of IPE, and questions how 'genuine' IPE can be achieved. In *Chapter 3*, Lyn Brown, a probation officer, debates further the issue of whether true integration takes place between health and social care, and argues that IPE has a valuable role to play in promoting workforce integration. She concludes that hard evidence needs to come from the practice setting, particularly with regard to the efficacy of coordinated packages of care to patients.

The allied health professions (AHPs) face specific challenges in implementing IPE, and this topic is clearly debated by Philip Turner in *Chapter 4*. He emphasises the crucial role taken by professional organisations and Workforce Development Confederations in support of IPE, and argues that AHPs need to play a greater leadership role in the NHS and become involved in the process of modernisation.

In chapter 5, Marilyn Hammick, who has a background in radiography, discusses the key issues that arise at all stages of the curriculum planning and approval process where IPE is part of a health or social care programme of education. This chapter will be indispensable for all those involved in preparation for a validation event where an IPE curriculum is meeting the needs of a number of healthcare professions.

Part 2 (Planning, implementing and evaluating IPE in practice) takes a clearly pragmatic stance, and provides details, from a variety of practice situations, of the various ways in which IPE is being implemented. These examples are underpinned by key strategic concepts in IPE, including team-building, collaboration and shared care. The value of understanding the role of others in the team, working effectively together and learning from colleagues feature significantly in Part 2. This part of the book aims to promote a greater understanding of IPE through examples of its implementation. In this way, readers can more effectively plan and implement IPE in their respective practice or education settings.

Part 2 begins with an exploration of conceptual and pragmatic issues arising from a multiprofessional communication skills training course. Tom Donovan, Dave Mercer and Ray Sutton present a case for the use of simulated patients in developing healthcare professionals' understanding of the patient's story (*Chapter 6*).

Chapter 7 provides an example of postgraduate IPE in the field of cancer and palliative care. Anne Lanceley offers a critique of the network agenda in this field and outlines an innovative educational programme that aims to help sustain attuned responses among professionals working with people who have cancer and who are dying. The programme will help healthcare professionals work with, and learn from, each other for the benefit of patients.

Chapter 8 continues the theme of team-working by arguing that progressive changes to routine practice are best effected through working with whole teams together, directly in the workplace. Mick McKeown and colleagues draw on two examples of this approach, and discuss projects based at Rathbone Hospital in Liverpool and Leigh Infirmary in Lancashire.

Helen Cooper is actively involved in teaching a wide variety of healthcare professionals; in *Chapter 9* she debates the very important issue of patient empowerment and the ways in which patients can be included in collaborative education and training. Using diabetes as the focus, she reviews current patterns of care and the importance of self-management, highlighting the need for a team approach to care and IPE.

Team-working is again reinforced in *Chapter 10*, where Tim Riding, who has a background in learning disabilities nursing, argues that this client group is likely to experience greater health need than its non-disabled counterpart. He argues that partnership is essential in this field and presents a strong case for the role of IPE in supporting this goal.

Chapter 11 focuses on primary care, and Kate Cernik and Caroline Carlisle explicitly address the benefits of IPE to community health. This chapter includes a number of case studies which describe some of the ways in which

IPE is being implemented, and helpfully outlines 'what worked well' and 'what was learned' from each of these studies.

Case studies are also a focus in *Chapter 12,* written by Di Marks-Maran and Gill Young from Thames Valley University. They describe two projects: one focuses on joint undergraduate work and the other looks at developing an online distance learning course in intensive care. A useful exploration of the potential of online programmes at a multiprofessional level is included.

In *Chapter 13,* Mike Farrell, a project manager in e-learning with a Workforce Development Confederation, sets out the potential for new learning technologies within the modernisation agenda.

The book concludes with a chapter that will help the reader reflect on some key issues in IPE. Written by Hugh Barr, Emeritus Professor of Interprofessional Education at the University of Westminster, *Chapter 14* explores the vital role that evaluation plays in IPE. Professor Barr asks some critical questions, which should guide individuals and organisations when evaluating IPE initiatives. We hope that readers of this book will take a critical view of the issues presented, and will find the debate stimulating. If readers are encouraged to identify ideas that they can transfer to their own clinical or educational field, then this book will have achieved its purpose.

Caroline Carlisle, Tom Donovan and Dave Mercer
April 2004

Department of Health (2000) *The NHS Plan. A plan for investment. A plan for reform.* The Stationery Office, London

Part 1

Interprofessional Education in Context

1

Towards a shared definition of interprofessional education

Caroline Carlisle, Tom Donovan and Dave Mercer

What is interprofessional education?

The scope and rapidity of change within the National Health Service in the past 20 years is unprecedented. Significant changes in healthcare practice, management and role development have shaped an NHS with vastly amended objectives from those of its original inception in 1946. By adopting new ways of working and extending and developing clinical roles, contemporary health care in the UK is now completely dependent upon multiprofessional approaches to care management and delivery.

Yet, despite these major changes in practice, formal educational preparation for health professionals remains largely uniprofessional. Although several initiatives appear to have yielded tangible improvements in some elements of learning (Foy *et al*, 2002; Wakefield *et al*, 2003), the statutory bodies responsible for shaping the learning agenda have neither imposed nor made significant moves towards developing a unified multiprofessional curriculum.

Part of the difficulty in establishing interprofessional education (IPE) arises from unclear, or sometimes conflicting, definitions of IPE. Terms such as 'shared learning', 'multiprofessional' and 'interprofessional' are used liberally and interchangeably in the literature, and appear to have some commonalities in meaning. Yet it remains difficult to find a term that accurately encompasses each. The World Health Organization (1988) defines multidisciplinary education as a process in which:

> '... students from health-related occupations, with different
> educational backgrounds, team together during certain periods of
> their education, with interaction as an important goal, to collaborate
> in providing promotive, preventive, curative, rehabilitative and other
> health-related services.'

A distinction between multiprofessional and interprofessional education is offered by Parsell and Bligh (1998), who contend that the term 'interprofessional' describes learning activities involving two professional groups, whereas 'multiprofessional' describes shared learning activities among three or more professional groups. Whichever term is used, the common theme of shared learning appears to be a consensual agreement that each represents a generic term for learning activities in which students from different spheres of health and social care coalesce within a framework of common learning aims and objectives.

Although IPE is not a 'new' educational concept, the current drive to develop multiprofessional approaches to care gained momentum in the light of recent scandals in health and social care settings in which health professionals failed to communicate adequately or were unaware of each other's activities and roles (Department of Health [DoH], 1999, 2003). A growing body of opinion appears to suggest that IPE may offer a solution to these issues through a potential – by shared learning activity – to improve professional relationships and ultimately enhance clinical care (Barrington *et al*, 1998; Carpenter, 1995).

The wider benefits of IPE also appear to influence and improve professional confidence, reflective practice, mutual professional respect and shared knowledge and skills (Munro *et al*, 2002). However, even within the context of an emerging evidence base in support of IPE, unanswered questions remain with regard to its appropriate place in curricula, its effectiveness compared with traditional educational models and its capacity to enhance or sustain learning.

Implicit within the nature of IPE is the acknowledgement that although health professionals may share common goals, specific expertise resides in exclusive areas of clinical practice. Given the growing evidence base within clinical specialties and the severe time constraints of clinical practice and educational activity, fundamental questions arise about the location of IPE opportunities in any professional curriculum. Even where apparent opportunities exist, role-specific issues within topics need to be addressed, and this presents challenges to educational providers, who may feel reluctant to 'dilute' an area of learning to accommodate multiprofessional perspectives.

Fundamental to any discussion about collaborative educational initiatives between different healthcare disciplines is the much-used, though often poorly understood, concept of 'power'. An astute observation is offered by Mintzberg and colleagues (1998: 264):

'Hold power up to a mirror and the reverse image you see is culture. Power takes that entity called organisation and fragments it: culture knits a collection of individuals into an integrated entity called organisation'.

The New Labour Government — emphasising inclusion, empowerment and citizenship — has chosen to focus on 'organisational culture' to promote a senbse of direction within the NHS. Educators need to be mindful of 'conflicting incentive structures' (Le Grand, 2002) and the 'rhetorical constructions of political realities' (Smith and Smith, 2000). Health policy is ideologically driven, and managers, practitioners and educators ought to engage critically with the language of health care – as rhetoric, jargon and metaphor (Richman and Mercer, 2003). The 'linguistic turn' of postmodern analyses (Lupton,

2001), and the work of Michel Foucault (1926–1984) in particular, hold tremendous vitality for understanding the relationship between knowledge and power through an exploration of discourse. Here, language is central to the way that we socially construct the world, and professional practice, through speaking and writing.

Hopefully, IPE has the potential to offer some degree of 'resistance' to the hierarchical dominance that has beleaguered professional equality in the workplace, and prioritised 'professional' ways of talking over 'patient' narratives. Achieving this is as much about sharing and clarifying values such as 'caring' and 'curing', as it is about the minutiae of 'swapping roles'.

Interprofessional developments in healthcare education and practice

The past few decades have witnessed increasing acceptance of the potential value and role of IPE within healthcare education. Much progress has been made since the days when multiprofessional education meant that disparate student groups were brought together simply for the purposes of managing scarce teaching resources and being able to deliver the same lecture to even more students at the same time. In recent years, a number of organisations have emerged that explicitly support quality IPE initiatives, e.g. the Learning and Teaching Support Network (LTSN), the UK Centre for the Advancement of Interprofessional Education (CAIPE).

It is gratifying to see that these organisations, among others, are exploring the evidence base for IPE. There is little doubt that the 'flavour of the month' criticism has been levied at the number of IPE initiatives that took place, justified purely on the feeling that it must be a good thing. There remains a lack of robust evidence for the effectiveness of IPE (Pirrie *et al*, 1999; Hammick, 2000) and it is to be hoped that there are now fewer educational innovations being conducted without concurrent evaluation research (Freeth *et al*, 2002).

The impetus for IPE initiatives has also come from recent healthcare policy statements advocating closer partnerships and cooperation between healthcare professionals, and also between health and social care agencies (DoH, 2000; Scottish Executive, 2001). The need to be more creative in meeting healthcare needs is essential at a time when professional staffing crises are occurring and there is evidence of growing numbers of unfilled posts in certain areas of NHS provision. Nursing shortages and the crisis in GP recruitment and retention, combined with increasing public expectations, mean that new ways must be found to provide a quality service. The new roles that many NHS staff are now taking on have often been created as part of an initial response to such issues as shortage of medical staff. Many of these new roles have been configured in unique and innovative ways and do not simply result in role substitution

(Woods, 2000). Without the commitment and collaboration of all members of the healthcare team, however, those developing or taking on these new roles will face unacceptable challenges during the change process. Designing IPE in such a way that professionals learn with and about each other can support the acceptance of flexible healthcare provision.

Patients still comment that they have difficulty in getting the specific help they need at the time they need it, partly because individual services do not seem to 'talk to each other' (Cooper *et al*, 2000). Effective interprofessional communication throughout the healthcare system is high on the policy agenda, not only among medical and nursing staff, but also among the allied health professions (AHP) workforce (Scottish Executive, 2003). The Government wants to give more power to frontline staff (DoH, 1999). This has a major impact on the way that working partnerships are developed across health and social care, and health professionals are finding that they must negotiate the delivery of their services with many new people (East, 2003).

The call for increasing flexibility between staff responsibilities and the need to break down traditional professional boundaries (DoH, 2002) mean that all staff must develop an understanding of the role and function of other members of the healthcare team. Without this, such issues as seamless care, team-working and appropriate referral mechanisms will be compromised. However, IPE is not a panacea: there may be additional, or indeed better, ways to achieve these targets.

Our expectations of what can be achieved through IPE must be realistic. It may not be essential that every IPE initiative meets the full spectrum of possible IPE outcomes. Objectives for IPE will vary according to a number of dimensions, such as whether it is delivered at pre-registration or post-registration level, whether it is focused on clinical skills or sharing values and beliefs, and whether it takes place in the workplace or an education institution. For example, a communication skills course for junior undergraduates can set objectives aimed at learning from each other and about each other's professional input in specific challenging situations. It may not, however, be necessary to have objectives in team-working outcomes at that early stage of education.

For IPE to be effective, however, it must address far more than simply shared learning. For example, it must involve patients in the design, teaching and assessment (Barr, 2001) and programmes should include group forming and maintenance components (Roberts *et al*, 2000). It should also promote an understanding, among students, of the underpinning values and aspirations of other professional groups (Salmon and Jones, 2000).

Caution is advised when identifying the benefits of IPE. Much of the current evidence focuses on the understanding of professional roles and team-working (Cooper *et al*, 2001) and stakeholder satisfaction (Barr *et al*, 2000). Students find IPE enjoyable and learn about other professionals' roles, although there can be many practical challenges such as large group sizes. Educators, too, enjoy IPE, but find issues around curricula modification and timetable clashes frustrating during the planning stages.

Few studies are adequately designed to measure whether the acquisition of knowledge and skills are affected by IPE. IPE study days held in a clinical skills laboratory for both medical and nursing students were positively evaluated, with medical students commenting on their increased understanding of holistic care, by Freeth and Chaput de Saintonge (2000). However, there is limited research on the potential effects of IPE conducted in practice settings. IPE has the potential to prepare students for the reality of interdisciplinary practice: evaluation research conducted on a training ward initiative found that students felt that the ward prepared them effectively for future practice (Reeves *et al*, 2002). Patients on this ward scored higher on a range of satisfaction indicators than a comparative group of patients. Few studies exist, however, which indicate whether IPE can benefit the direct care of patients and clients through clinical outcome measures.

Does IPE have an effect on interprofessional team-working?

Given the predominance of favourable accounts of IPE within the literature, and even accounting for the absence of a substantive, supporting evidence base, superficially it is easy to assume an implicit connection between IPE and improved team-working. However, as health professionals continue to struggle with surmounting a perceived theory–practice gap in traditional educational programmes, practitioners and educators should approach such assumptions with caution. Long experience shows that educational activities do not always translate into effective practice, and it is therefore unwise to assume that IPE will fare any more successfully than traditional and well-established approaches. IPE remains primarily a different process of organising educational activity rather than offering a new way of learning, where the idea of team working is far from unproblematic.

Kemp (2003) locates the concept of 'team', historically and cross-culturally, within an array of meanings and metaphors. This analysis corresponds to the Freudian notion of a 'multiplex metaphor', collapsing a whole series of ideas and interpretations into a single entity. In addition to the widely cited definition of 'team', which typically informs healthcare rhetoric, as 'a set of persons working together...' (*Concise Oxford Dictionary*, 1983), it further connotes a multiplicity of images which have resonance for policy and practice. 'Team' can therefore also describe 'beasts of burden' harnessed together in the performance of drudgery, or the competitive spirit of the 'sporting' domain – appropriate to the market economy. Similarly, within the primary care setting, practitioners drawing upon a 'sexual' metaphor found team to be an unsatisfactory term to the extent that it was represented by a pattern of domination. Thus, if the jargon of team-working presents an image of commonality and striving towards shared goals, the ideal of equality is compromised by the reality of captaincy, leadership and superiority mediated by medical power in general practice (Kemp, 2003).

A woefully tiresome and commonplace expression in managerial parlance impels us to 'sing from the same hymn sheet'. With this cliché in mind, it is important that any attempts to utilise IPE recognise the political naivety of seeing the healthcare team as an 'orchestra', each member playing a different instrument but united in the quest for harmony. Again, a more meaningful and critical engagement with the issues is afforded by the insights of postmodernity, where the organisation exists only as a series of people linked together by ideas and imagery. Shifting models of management within the organisational structure of the NHS have produced a fundamental conflict between bureaucracy (universal laws) and professionalism (accountability) played out on a 'ritualistic battleground'.

It is suggested that the healthcare system in the UK never generated organisational theory (Richman, 1987). Historically, decision-making resided in autonomous clinical specialists where the hospital represented a negotiated social order – perfectly captured in consultants referring to 'my patients' and 'my beds'. Here, leadership is premised upon the theoretical foundation of medical knowledge as paradigmatic, dynamic and changing over time (Jewson, 1976). In contrast, the contemporary managerial culture of budgetary control, performance indicators and audit comprises a collection of untested practices where clinical expertise is overshadowed by the dictates of the resource base. The relevance of this critique to IPE finds expression in the possibility of inter-disciplinary practice as free-floating and open to debate within an inflexible structure of 'high command' management.

Conclusions

The future role of IPE in healthcare is uncertain, but holds promise for creativity and innovation in preparing a new generation of professionals, where a spirit of egalitarianism can prosper. To this extent, ideally IPE will meet the demands of contemporary health policy and education. However, implementation of the IPE ideal in practice presents a number of conceptual and pragmatic challenges. Many of these challenges are debated by the contributors to this book. Although their individual experiences and perspectives differ, all share a commitment and enthusiasm to the delivery of a 'first-class service' and exploring the ways that IPE can contribute to this agenda.

References

Barr H (2001) *Interprofessional Education. Today, yesterday and tomorrow.* A review commissioned by LTSN/CAIPE, London

Barr H, Freeth D, Hammick M, Koppel I, Reeves S (2000) *Evaluations of Interprofessional Education: A UK review for health and social care.* CAIPE/BERA, London

Barrington D, Rodger M, Gray L, Jones B, Landridge M, Marriot R (1998) Student evaluation of an interactive, multidisciplinary clinical learning model. *Med Teach* **20**: 530–5

Carpenter J (1995) Interprofessional education for medical and nursing students: evaluation of a programme. *Med Educ* **29**; 265–72

Cooper H, Carlisle C, Gibbs T, Watkins C (2000) *Interprofessional Education: An exploration of its potential for the training of undergraduate health professionals.* University of Liverpool, Liverpool

Cooper H, Carlisle C, Gibbs T, Watkins C (2001) Developing an evidence base for interdisciplinary learning: a systematic review. *J Adv Nurs* **35**(2): 228–37

Department of Health (1999) *The Report of the Committee of Inquiry into the Personality Disorder Unit, Ashworth Special Hospital* (The Fallon Inquiry Report). Cm 4194–11. The Stationery Office, London

Department of Health (2000) *The NHS Plan. A plan for investment. A plan for reform.* The Stationery Office, London

Department of Health (2002) *Liberating the Talents: Helping primary care trusts and nurses to deliver the NHS Plan.* Department of Health, London

Department of Health (2003) *The Victoria Climbié Inquiry* (The Lord Laming Report). The Stationery Office, London

East K (2003) Voicepiece. *AHP Bulletin* **15**: 2l. Department of Health, London

Freeth DS, Chaput de Saintonge DM (2000) Helping medical students become good house officers: interprofessional learning in a skills centre. *Medical Teacher* **22**(4): 392–8

Freeth D, Hammick M, Koppel I, Reeves S, Barr H (2002) *A Critical Review of Evaluations of Interprofessional Education.* CAIPE, London

Foy R, Tidy N, Hollis S (2002) Interprofessional learning form primary care: lessons from an action learning programme. *Br J Clin Governance* **7**(1): 40–4

Hammick M (2000) IPE: evidence from the past to guide the future. *Med Teach* **22**: 472–8

Jewson N (1976) The disappearance of the sick-man from medical cosmology. 1770–870 *Sociology* **10**: 225–44

Kemp LJ (2003) Organisational teams: modern and postmodern perspectives in primary healthcare. Unpublished PhD thesis, Manchester Metropolitan University, Manchester

Le Grand J (2002) The Labour Government and the National Health Service. *Oxford Review of Economic Policy* **18**(2): 137–53

Lupton D (2001) *Medicine as Culture: Illness, Disease and the Body in Western Societies*. Sage, London

Mintzberg H, Ahlstrand B, Lampel J (1998) *Strategy Safari*. Pearson Education, Harlow: 264

Munro N, Felton A, McIntosh C (2002) Is multidisciplinary learning effective among those caring for people with diabetes? *Diabet Med* **19**: 799–803

Parsell G, Bligh J (1998) Interprofessional learning. *Postgrad Med J* **74**: 89–95

Pirrie A, Hamilton S, Wilson V (1999) Multidisciplinary education: some issues and concerns. *Educ Res* **41**; 301–14

Reeves S, Freeth D, McCrorie P, Perry D (2002) 'It teaches you what to expect in future…': interprofessional learning on a training ward for medical, nursing, occupational therapy and physiotherapy students. *Med Educ* **36**(4): 337–44

Richman J (1987) *Medicine and Health*. Longman, London

Richman J, Mercer D (2004) 'Modern language' or 'spin'?: 'newspeak' and organisational culture. *J Nurs Manag* (in press)

Roberts C, Howe A, Winterburn S, Fox N (2000) Not so easy as it sounds: a qualitative study of a shared learning project between medical and nursing undergraduate students. *Med Teach* **22**(4): 386–91

Salmon D, Jones M (2001) Shaping the interprofessional agenda: a study examining qualified nurses' perceptions of learning with others. *Nurse Educ Today* **21**: 18–25

Scottish Executive (2001) *Caring for Scotland: The strategy for nursing and midwifery in Scotland*. The Stationery Office, Edinburgh

Scottish Executive (2003) *Building on Success: Future directions for the allied health professions in Scotland*. The Stationery Office, Edinburgh

Smith CA, Smith KB (2000) A rhetorical perspective on the 1997 British party manifestos. *Political Communication* **17**: 457–73

Wakefield A, Furber C, Boggis C, Sutton A, Cooke S (2003) Promoting interdisciplinarity through educational initiative: a qualitative evaluation. *Nurse Educ Pract* **3**: 195–203

Woods LP (2000) *The Enigma of Advanced Nursing Practice*. Quay Books, a division of MA Healthcare Limited, Dinton, Wiltshire

World Health Organization (1988) *Learning Together to Work Together for Health*. Report of a WHO study group on multiprofessional education of health personnel. World Health Organization Technical Report Series 769. WHO, Geneva

2

The education and practice agenda for interprofessional teaching and learning

Sally Gosling

The concept of interprofessional education (IPE) has become more topical in recent years: it is now prominent in learning and teaching strategies for preparing future healthcare professionals for practice and for meeting the ongoing learning needs of qualified staff. This chapter addresses a series of linked questions related to IPE and practice:

- what is the interprofessional agenda and what are its drivers?
- what are the goals of IPE?
- how can genuine IPE be achieved?
- what are the barriers, threats and limitations?

Current agenda and policy drivers

IPE is not new, with several surveys highlighting a variety of initiatives over the last two decades (Horder, 1992; Barr and Waterton, 1996; Barr *et al*, 1999; Zwarenstein *et al*, 1999; Barr *et al*, 2000; Zwarenstein *et al*, 2002). However, the agenda surrounding IPE has recently gained new vigour:

- it now has a greater number of advocates and followers
- it is informed by increasingly sophisticated ideas about what it should involve
- it enjoys greater clarity on what its aims should be, matched by a more questioning approach to how — and whether — these can be achieved
- more resources and stronger professional, academic and political will should underpin its integration into healthcare education at all levels if declared intent is carried forward.

A growing emphasis on the need for IPE, and a more genuine shift to interprofessional practice, are linked strongly to government initiatives to modernise patient care. This broad agenda has many strands. These have been rehearsed and developed in a number of documents (Department of Health [DoH], 2000; Scottish Executive, 2000; Bristol Royal Infirmary Enquiry [BRI], 2001; Department of Health, Social Services and Public Safety [DHSSPS],

2001; National Assembly for Wales, 2001; British Medical Association [BMA] Health Policy and Economic Research Unit, 2002; Department of Health and Universities UK [DoH and UUK], 2002; DoH, 2002; Wanless, 2002). In summary, the key goals are:

- to enhance quality of care
- to better respond to patient need
- greater user involvement
- improved consistency
- increased capacity (supported by enlarged financial resources)
- better integration of services and sectors
- greater efficiency.

IPE is just one element in realising these goals. However, it carries a heavy symbolism in terms of changing working practices and workforce planning (Humphris and Macleod Clark, 2002) and professional relationships and responsibilities (Salvage, 2002).

Until recently, a genuine commitment to IPE seems to have been held by relatively few, with such an approach appearing to present too great a challenge to professions and too many practical difficulties to potential providers (Hutt, 1980; Goble, 1994; Shaw, 1994). Now it has become established thinking in healthcare education, forming a definite aspiration of most. The increased enthusiasm for both IPE and interprofessional practice is premised on the need for health and social care practitioners to collaborate with one another and, just as importantly, with the patients and clients they serve (Hornby and Atkins, 2000; Kendall, 2001). The emphasis is therefore on healthcare professionals developing a mutual understanding of one another (WHO, 1988), an awareness of the need for collaboration (Hutt, 1980), and the skills to collaborate effectively (Centre for the Advancement of Interprofessional Education [CAIPE], 1997).

We seem to be moving away, then, from IPE as a 'vague concept,' towards the 'critical mass' needed to establish interprofessional learning and teaching firmly within provision (Goble, 1994). In short, the 'compelling logic' that those 'who will practise together should be educated together' is now widely acknowledged (Patti and Hentschke, 1998). What is still for debate – and to be proved – is how IPE can best be delivered and how its positive impact on practice can be demonstrated. The agenda is complex, hinging on long-term, cultural change for its realisation. As Hugh Barr (2002) has observed, IPE forms an 'unfinished fabric'.

The goals of IPE

Unsurprisingly, there are contradictory and conflicting ideas about IPE. These reflect the different complexion put upon what it should be about. For some time the term was used simply to indicate a style of provision primarily motivated by economies of scale and covering subject areas for students from different professional groups (Horder, 1992). This rather loose usage has more recently been resisted. Primacy is now given to IPE being concerned with developing the attributes, skills and values required for effective team-working and genuinely patient-centred care (Miller *et al*, 2001).

If anything, this issue has become more complicated by two, related government initiatives in England: focused encouragement of IPE, and the promotion, which may well become a condition of education commissioning, of strands of common curricula across healthcare provision (NHS Executive [NHSE], 2001; DoH & UUK, 2002). While these are undoubtedly linked, they are not the same: the former recognises the need to cultivate the aptitude and skills required for collaborative working, while the latter acknowledges healthcare students' shared learning needs (Barr, 2002). Benchmark statements can perhaps help to chart a way through needs in both areas, as explored later.

Fundamental questions have to be asked about IPE, particularly when its application is being urged so heavily. Is IPE really needed and does it achieve its goals? Answers to these questions are closely aligned. The need for IPE is based on the changes in healthcare delivery summarised above, and the growing recognition that those preparing to become, and practising as, healthcare professionals must work together to serve patients' needs effectively, efficiently and sensitively.

The natural link between IPE and equipping participants for collaboration has been made for some time (Areskog, 1988). However, recent studies have highlighted that, despite heavy rhetoric and assumptions, there is no tangible evidence of IPE's effectiveness (Zwarenstein *et al*, 1999; Koppel *et al*, 2001; Barr, 2002; Zwarenstein *et al*, 2002). But this lack of affirmation cannot be taken as evidence that IPE does not work. Moreover, the varying aims and approaches of initiatives to date cloud the search for proof of effectiveness. As many have not been concerned with developing the attributes required of collaborative practice, it is unfair to subject them to an evaluation of whether they have succeeded in doing this. It is for new studies, including those that can comply with the rigour required by Cochrane Library reviews, to demonstrate the worth of IPE activities, of which the espoused aim is to nurture collaboration (Zwarenstein *et al*, 2002).

The intended, albeit implicit, goal of IPE is perceived as breaking down existing professional identities. At its extreme this goal is seen as creating new practitioners whose scope of activity is defined along quite different lines from, and whose province of skills and knowledge might be significantly broader than, current healthcare professionals (Oxford Regional Health Authority, 1995; University of Manchester, 1996). Such a perceived intent poses a threat to IPE becoming embedded in pedagogical approaches. While radical change to professional role configuration may be the covert and, in some cases, explicit aspiration of some, this is not what IPE is about (Barr, 2002; Zwarenstein *et al*, 2002).

The difference between IPE and blurring the distinctions between different professional groups to the extent that they cease to exist needs to be acknowledged by policy makers, education commissioners and providers and healthcare regulators. A firm, coherent relationship has to be maintained between education, job role and regulation if public safety is to be preserved. A balance has therefore to be struck between professional roles being sufficiently flexible to respond to service needs and their being sustained by a defined knowledge, skills and evidence base and appropriate regulatory processes. IPE and interprofessional practice have to be taken forward with this firmly in mind if their goals are to be fulfilled. At the same time, account has to be taken of the trend towards creating new sub-professional roles, for example, assistant practitioners whose scope of practice relates to patient care pathways, such as alongside radiographers. There are also shifts in the roles of existing professions, which can be supported by the development of foundation degrees (Greater Manchester Workforce Development Confederation, 2002; Humphris and Macleod Clark, 2002; McGauran, 2002).

Barriers, threats and limitations

The barriers, threats and limitations to IPE and interprofessional practice are multifaceted. They can be categorised as either an issue of perceptions and attitudes, or of matters of organisation and resources (Connelly, 1978; Carpenter, 1989; Casto, 1994; Goble 1994).

There comes a point when the two simply meld. If there is not a will, there is unlikely to be a way, while those responsible for educating current and future members of the healthcare professions cannot be expected to implement interprofessional learning and teaching strategies if the structures in which they work militate against this. Until recently, individual healthcare programmes have often been physically distant from one another, offered in different geographical locations and/or provided by different institutions. The almost wholesale integration of healthcare education into the university sector – along with the increasing expectation that universities work in partnership with one another and with the further education sector – should provide a more promising basis for developments (Barr, 2002; DoH and UUK, 2002; Higgs and Edwards, 2002). However, there is still a need for real intent and practical measures. Consideration is given to the barriers, threats and limitations to IPE, along with potential ways of addressing these in the sections below.

Structures and practicalities

Coordinating and synchronising interprofessional learning sessions can present challenges that might be deemed insuperable, particularly when the amassed cohorts from different healthcare programmes represent sizeable student numbers. In particular, the sequencing and length of practice-based learning components is a barrier to bringing students together, especially where attempts are made to attend to the needs of cohorts from a variety of established routes and, possibly, from different institutions (Freeth *et al*, 2001). This is an aim within a number of the current pilot initiatives to modernise qualifying education within the allied health professions. It is also a strong implication within proposals to streamline and make more equitable the respective funding structures in healthcare education (NHSE, 2001; DoH & UUK, 2002). It will be important to follow the progress of these.

To compound matters, it is sometimes claimed that it is not higher education institutions themselves that inhibit creative curriculum design and timetabling, but the professional and statutory regulatory bodies that validate provision (Weinstein, 1994). It is all too easy to reach stalemate if such perceptions persist. However, none is necessarily well founded. Opportunities for progress to be made are signalled by:

- developments occurring in professional healthcare regulation (Health Professions Council, 2002)
- professional bodies' increasing enthusiasm to work together on common issues (Chartered Society of Physiotherapy [CSP], 2002a,b)
- growing awareness across agencies that approval processes have to change if they are to be receptive to workforce demands (Shaw, 1994).

What is needed, if progress is to be made, is a more lateral approach to curriculum design, programme structuring and fulfilling programme approval requirements. In short, structures and funding streams have to accommodate and reflect the full implications of IPE.

There is increasing recognition of the need to deploy practical approaches to IPE if students are to develolp the skills required for collaboration and team-working and to see this as worthwhile (Evans, 1991; Weinstein, 1994; Miller *et al*, 2001). Students need to be encouraged, through exposure to interprofessional practice-based learning, to see working collaboratively with colleagues, and with patients and carers, as fundamental to their professional practice, rather than something peripheral (McCroskey, 1998; Freeth *et al*, 2001). Problem-based learning enmeshed firmly in practice seems promising, provided that appropriate changes are made to institutional structures and processes to accommodate this (Hutt, 1980; Savin-Baden, 2000; Freeth *et al*, 2001).

Nurturing identity

Developing mutual understanding of different professionals' roles and individuals' capacity for patient-focused collaboration raises fundamental questions, including:

- what is the nature of professional identity (Salvage, 2002)?
- what are the concepts of professionalism (Davies, 1996)?
- how can attributes related to these be nurtured and developed (Hornby and Atkins, 2000)?

At its most basic, individuals need to be sufficiently secure in their professional identity (albeit nascent in the case of prequalifying students) not to feel threatened by learning with others. There are not only different perspectives on how professional identity is forged and the relationship between this and readiness for learning with and about others, but also contrasting views about the most appropriate timing of IPE. How far is it feasible, valuable and necessary to include interprofessional learning within qualifying education programmes?

Students might be assumed to lack sufficient confidence in their professional identity to cope with learning that has working relationships with colleagues on other study routes as a significant component. Conversely, it seems almost irresponsible to assume that it is safe for students not to gain some interprofessional learning experience before qualifying, because, as newly qualified practitioners, they will work as members of multiprofessional teams. To do this effectively, they have to understand others' roles and appreciate how respective profession-specific contributions need to fit into a seamless whole (Quality Assurance Agency [QAA], 2001; CSP, 2002a; QAA, 2002a). No longer, then, can interprofessional learning be seen as optional within qualifying programmes. Rather, it forms an essential prerequisite for future professional practice (BRI, 2001; NHSE, 2001; DoH and UUK, 2002). At the same time, approaches need to be sensitive to participants' stage of professional development and to involve students at broadly similar stages, for example, in terms of their previous exposure to practice settings (Loxley, 1997; Miller *et al*, 2001).

Bringing together students who present significantly different levels of academic attainment and presumed capacity for ongoing learning presents a challenge. It might be deemed too difficult to develop learning opportunities for diverse student groups, accommodating, for example, medical students presenting high levels of academic achievement and fulfilling standard entry patterns to higher education and those from other professional routes, such as nursing, who present much more varying academic, experience and age profiles. However, perceiving a difficulty in creating mixed cohorts negates the possibilities for approaches that capitalise on common experience, understanding and learning needs, as well as the value of students learning from one another (Hornby and Atkins, 2000). As McCroskey (1998) observed:

'Personality and maturity of individual students are more important than their educational status.'

Student attitudes

Students' receptiveness to IPE is an essential ingredient for success (Parsell and Bligh, 1999). Studies suggest that student attitudes can vary quite markedly, with some participants perceiving that they have less to gain from shared learning than their peers from other student groups and seeing IPE as an unhelpful distraction from their profession-specific studies (Horsburgh *et al*, 2001). This relates to fixed, often hierarchical, ideas about the knowledge and skills base of different professions (Hornby and Atkins, 2000). It can also reflect received views on the relative status of each profession and stereotyping that shapes individuals' thinking about healthcare practice from the outset of their qualifying education (Horsburgh *et al*, 2001; Salvage, 2002).

There is a danger that IPE initiatives can actually reinforce such stereotyping (Pearson *et al*, 1985; Carpenter, 1989; Goble, 1994; Carpenter and Hewstone, 1996). This affirms the need to develop students' understanding of different professional groups' contribution to patient care and their capacity to work across professional boundaries. Strategies are needed to raise awareness of the importance of IPE, including those that revolve around problem-based and placement learning, so that students and qualified practitioners come to recognise the value of collaboration and of genuinely developing an understanding of one another (McCroskey, 1998; Miller *et al*, 2001; Savin-Baden, 2000).

Post-qualifying learning and development

It is perhaps easily assumed that IPE has been more successfully integrated into post-qualifying education than into qualifying programmes, not least because issues of security of professional identity should not apply (Areskog, 1988; Horder, 1992). In reality, much of what has formed interprofessional continuing professional development (CPD) provision has simply been about using available resources expediently, matching supply with demand and making available learning experiences that can valuably be accessed by different professions.

Given the reality of recruitment, what might have been intended as a learning opportunity for a range of professions and as offering scope for professionals to share their knowledge, skills, experience and perspectives can become heavily skewed to one profession. For example, a programme designed to cater for the CPD needs of nurses and physiotherapists in an area such as palliative care may attract participants in far greater numbers from the former, simply because of their greater presence in the workforce. It seems reasonable to suppose, therefore, that post-qualifying education has to develop as much as qualifying education if it is truly to promote interprofessional learning that nurtures shared respect and understanding and develops the attributes required for collaboration (DoH, 2001; Miller *et al*, 2001).

Moving forward

Benchmark statements, prepared under the aegis of the Quality Assurance Agency for Higher Education, offer a potentially promising way forward for promoting IPE. Within nursing, midwifery, health visiting and the allied health professions, an 'emerging framework' has been distilled from profession-specific statements that rehearses key qualities and attributes (QAA, 2001). Parallel benchmark statements developed for medicine contain similar elements (QAA, 2002a).

A process of mapping, perhaps with two central foci on developing students' capacity for interprofessional, collaborative working and equipping students with the common attributes required for patient-focused care, could help higher education institutions review their curricula to optimise opportunities for shared learning in preparing students for the changing demands of healthcare.

Table 2.1 highlights key elements from both QAA documents, which might form the focus of such an exercise. Identifying the scope for streamlining academic, professional and regulatory requirements across professional routes, along with integrating QAA programme specifications firmly into programme development, might be a further way of making the significant task of successful IPE that much easier (QAA, 2002b).

Conclusion

IPE should aim to instil the values, attributes and skills required of team-working, and have as its focus the efficient delivery of patient-centred, evidence-based care of a consistently high quality. There is a need to raise awareness that the interdependent nature of professions' contributions does not undermine individuals' roles, but is essential to serving patient needs (Patti and Hentschke, 1998). Perhaps the greatest threat to IPE becoming established firmly within provision is that it has still to prove it can fulfil these aims.

An increasingly refined and shared understanding of the goals of IPE should, in time, manifest in rigorous approaches and evaluative studies that can attest to the effectiveness of learning and teaching strategies at both qualifying and post-qualifying levels (Koppel *et al*, 2001; Zwarenstein *et al*, 2002). It is important that evaluations of initiatives are disseminated and used to inform future approaches across higher education institutions and geographical regions. Good practice needs to be shared (CAIPE, 1997). Lessons need to be learned from exploratory exercises and effective approaches embedded in institutional, staffing and regulatory structures and recognition schemes (McCroskey, 1998).

Table 2.1: Elements summarised from benchmark statements

Interprofessional learning needs

❖ Ability to work with other healthcare professionals, recognising the contribution of each

❖ Effective team-working centred on delivering best service to patients

❖ Interprofessional/inter-agency approaches to health and social care

❖ Interpersonal skills relating to effective communication with patients, carers and colleagues

Common learning needs

❖ NHS organisation and cross-sector working

❖ Recognising limits of professional competence and exercising professional judgement

❖ Appropriate professional behaviours

❖ Ethical, legal and professional responsibilities

❖ Principles of patient partnership

❖ Care planning

❖ Educating others

Source: QAA, 2001, 2002a

It would be wrong to assume either that there is one way to deliver IPE or that IPE offers a panacea for achieving a perfect match between healthcare education and fulfilling service needs. However, it should aid progress if it is accompanied by strategies that enable students to:

- acquire profession-specific knowledge, skills and attributes
- use and develop the evidence base critically
- develop a commitment to career-long learning and development
- understand the responsibilities and privileges that professional status confers

- engage in delivering health care that is genuinely centred on patient partnership and empowerment.

With this caveat, and accepting that many of the above can, in part, be addressed through shared learning, the ultimate test for IPE is whether it translates into practice where duplication is minimised, quality is maximised and the contributions of individual practitioners, patients and carers to fulfilling common, shared goals are genuinely respected and valued.

References

Areskog NH (1988) The need for multiprofessional health education in undergraduate studies. *Med Educ* **22**: 251–2

Barr H (2002) *Interprofessional Education Today, Yesterday and Tomorrow.* Occasional Paper No.1. Centre for Health Sciences and Practice (Learning and Teaching Support Network). King's College, London

Barr H, Waterton S (1996) *Interprofessional Education in Health and Social Care in the United Kingdom.* Report of a CAIPE Survey. Centre for the Advancement of Interprofessional Education, London

Barr H, Hammick M, Koppel I, Reeves S (1999) Evaluating IPE: Two systematic reviews for health and social care. *Br Educ Res J* **25**(4): 533–44

Barr H, Freeth D, Hammick M, Koppel I, Reeves S (2000) *Evaluations of Interprofessional Education.* Centre for the Advancement of Interprofessional Education with the British Educational Research Association, London

Bristol Royal Infirmary (2001) Final Report. *Learning from Bristol: The Report of the Public Inquiry in Children's Heart Surgery at the Bristol Royal Infirmary 1984– 1995* Command paper: CM5207. BRI Inquiry, Bristol

British Medical Association Health Policy and Economic Research Unit (2002) *The Future Healthcare Workforce.* Discussion Paper 9. BMA, London

Carpenter J (1989) Interprofessional education. *Primary Healthcare* **July**: 21

Carpenter J, Hewstone M (1996) Shared learning for doctors and social workers: evaluation of a programme. *British Journal of Social Work* **26**: 239–57

Casto M (1994) Interprofessional work in the USA — education and practice. In: Leathard A (Ed). *Going Interprofessional: Working together for health and welfare.* Routledge, London: 188–205

Centre for the Advancement of Interprofessional Education (CAIPE) (1997) Interprofessional education: what, how and when? *CAIPE Bulletin* **13**: 19

Chartered Society of Physiotherapy (2002a) *Curriculum Framework for Qualifying Programmes in Physiotherapy.* CSP, London

Chartered Society of Physiotherapy (2002b) *Allied Health Professions: Value statement on future arrangements for the approval of qualifying programmes under the Health Professions Council.* CSP, London

Connelly T Jr (1978) Basic organisational considerations for interdisciplinary education development in the health sciences. *J Allied Health* **7**(4): 274–80

Davies C (1996) A new vision of professionalism. *Nurs Times* **13**(92): 54–6

Department of Health (2000) *The NHS Plan. A plan for investment. A plan for reform.* The Stationery Office, London

Department of Health (2001) *Working Together — Learning Together. A framework for lifelong learning in the NHS.* DoH, London

Department of Health (2002) *Delivering the NHS Plan: Next steps on investment, next steps on reform.* DoH, London

Department of Health, Social Services and Public Safety (DHSSPS) (2001) *Best Practice — Best Care. A framework for setting standards, delivering services and improving monitoring and regulation of the HPSS.* A Consultation Paper. DHSSPS, Belfast

Department of Health & Universities UK (DoH & UUK) (2002) *Funding Learning and Development for the Healthcare Workforce.* DoH, London

Evans S (1991) Interdisciplinary Learning. *Postgraduate Education for General Practice* **2**: 41–7

Freeth D, Reeves S, Goreham C, Parker P, Haynes S, Pearson S (2001) 'Real life' clinical learning on an interprofessional training ward. *Nurse Educ Today* **21**: 366–72

Goble R (1994) Multi-professional education in Europe. An overview. In: Leathard A (Ed). *Going Interprofessional: Working together for health and welfare.* Routledge, London: 175–87

Greater Manchester Workforce Development Confederation (2002) *Delivering the Workforce.* WDC, Greater Manchester

Health Professions Council (2002) *The Future. A paper for consultation.* HPC, London

Higgs J, Edwards H (2002) Challenges facing health professional education in the changing context of university education. *Br J Occup Ther* **65**(7): 315–20

Horder P (1992) A national survey that needs to be repeated. *J Interprof Care* **6**(1): 65–71

Hornby S, Atkins J (2000) *Collaborative Care: Interprofessional, Interagency, Interpersonal.* Blackwell Science, Oxford

Horsburgh M, Lamdin R, Williamson E (2001) Multiprofessional learning: the attitudes of medical, nursing and pharmacy students to shared learning. *Med Educ* **35**: 876–83

Humphris D, Macleod Clark J (2002) *Shaping a Vision for a 'New Generation' Workforce.* Future Health Worker Project. Institute for Public Policy Research, London

Hutt A (1980) Shared learning for shared care. *J Adv Nurs* **5**: 389–96

Kendall L (2001) *The Future Patient.* Institute for Public Policy Research, London

Koppel I, Barr H, Reeves S, Freeth D, Hammick M (2001) Establishing a systematic approach to evaluating the effectiveness of interprofessional education. *Issues in Interdisciplinary Care* **3**(1):41–9

Loxley A (1997) *Collaboration in Health and Welfare: Working with Difference.* Jessica Kingsley, London

McCroskey J (1998) Remaking professional and interprofessional education. In: McCroskey J, Einbinder SD (Eds). *Universities and Communities: Remaking Professional and Inter-professional Education for the Next Century.* Praeger: 3–24

McGauran A (2002) Doctoring the usual roles. *Health Serv J* **112**:14–15

Miller C, Freeman M, Ross N (2001) *Interprofessional Practice in Health and Social Care: Challenging the Shared Learning Agenda.* Arnold, London

National Assembly of Wales (2001) *Improving Health in Wales — A plan for the NHS with its partners.* National Assembly of Wales, Cardiff

NHS Executive(NHSE) (2001) *Modernising Pre-registration Education for the Allied Health Professions: Physiotherapy, occupational therapy, radiography (diagnostic and/or therapeutic) and chiropody/podiatry.* NHSE, London

Oxford Regional Health Authority (1995) *The Education and Training of Rehabilitation Therapists.* Oxford RHA, Oxford

Parsell G, Bligh J (1999) The development of a questionnaire to assess the readiness of healthcare students for inter-professional learning (RIPLS). *Med Educ* **33**: 95–100

Patti RJ, Hentschke G (1998) Professional and interprofessional perspectives. In: McCroskey J, Einbinder SD (Eds). *Universities and Communities: Remaking professional and inter-professional education for the next century.* Praeger, Connecticut: 257–67

Pearson L, Morris P, Whitehouse C (1985) Consumer-oriented groups: a new approach to interdisciplinary teaching. *J R Coll Gen Pract* **35**: 381–3

Quality Assurance Agency (2001) *Benchmark Statement: Healthcare Programmes.* QAA, Gloucester

Quality Assurance Agency (2002a) *Medicine: Benchmark Statement.* QAA, Gloucester

Quality Assurance Agency (2002b) *Guidelines for Preparing Programme Specifications.* QAA, Gloucester

Salvage J (2002) *Rethinking Professionalism: The first step for patient-focused care?* Future Health Worker Project. Institute for Public Policy Research, London

Savin-Baden M (2000) *Problem-based Learning in Higher Education: Untold stories.* Society for Research into Higher Education and Open University Press, Buckingham

Scottish Executive (2000) *Our National Health: A plan for action, a plan for change.* Scottish Executive, Edinburgh

Shaw I (1994) *Evaluating Interprofessional Training.* Avebury, Aldershot

University of Manchester (1996) *The Future Healthcare Workforce.* University of Manchester, Manchester

Wanless D (2002) *Securing Our Future Health: Taking a long-term view.* The Public Enquiry Office, London

Weinstein J (1994) *Sewing the Seams for a Seamless Service. A review of developments in interprofessional education and training.* Central Council for the Education and Training of Social Workers, London

World Health Organization (1988) *Learning Together to Work Together for Health.* WHO, Geneva

Zwarenstein M, Atkins J, Barr H, Hammick M, Reeves S (1999) A systematic review of interprofessional education, *J Interprof Care* **13**(4): 417-24

Zwarenstein M, Reeves S, Barr H, Hammick M, Koppel I, Atkins J (2004) *Interprofessional Education: Effects on professional practice and health care outcomes* (Cochrane Review). In: The Cochrane Library, Issue 2, Oxford

3

The integration of health and social care: myth or reality?

Lyn Brown

More than thirty years ago I was one of the first female probation officers to begin working in a large all-male prison. The challenges of 'survival' in this position were numerous. Not least was the core issue of maintaining a professional identity and practice role, which was no longer autonomous, combined with managing the confidentiality of probation records. Prison officers who had their own occupational culture, networks and routines (Fitzgerald and Sim, 1982) were suddenly expected to work alongside a group of professionals whom they had previously viewed as 'softies' or 'do-gooders'. The allocation of prison keys and office space to probation staff added to the sense of discomfort.

Short joint residential courses, in comfortable settings, were designed to help integration of the two organisations. This initiative ran throughout the 1980s and into the 1990s. Not everything could be 'thrashed out' in these sessions. However, the use of prison humour through film and role play relaxed participants sufficiently to allow the expression of honest opinions about working practice, a review of the aims of prison work and, finally, ways forward. Mixed pairings of participants were allocated project work to be undertaken between the two separate residential weeks. An evaluation of the programme revealed increased knowledge and understanding of the work that others performed, enhanced cooperation — especially where participants came from the same institution — and improved understanding of the penal and probation services.

Following a reorganisation of training, these courses ceased operating in the mid-1990s. In January 2002, an Offender Assessment System (OASys), shared by the prison and probation services, was presented as a 'prototype'. Service circulars (National Probation Directorate Circulars PC 16 2002 and PC 22 2002) indicated a problem regarding 'identification of a single view between the prison and probation services of the sensitivity of the information used in OASys'. The 'lesson' here is that short courses may well effect changes, but if these are to be sustained other structures and strategies need to be put into place. Reflecting on this early experience of 'joint education' is an interesting starting point for exploration of the contemporary role of interprofessional education (IPE) in the context of health and social care. This chapter looks at some of the issues that need to be addressed if integration is to be implemented and sustained.

Defining health and social care

The question has been posed in undergraduate seminars: 'What has social care to do with real doctoring?' The answer lies in the fact that an illness, disability or accident that happens to a body is also experienced by the person inhabiting that body. Modern medicine recognises this and integrates the traditional biomedical model with a psychosocial and economic perspective in the diagnosis of health problems, thus providing wider options for patient care. If we recognise this integration in diagnosis, it follows that treatment plans also need to integrate health care with social care. Policy can help or hinder the process of collaboration, but rivalries and misconceptions between those involved in health care also play their part.

The first issue is one of definition. It is easy to be confused by the numerous definitions of health and social care that exist in the literature or find expression during meetings between various professional groups. We are all guilty of using acronyms and exclusive words, and it is easy to assume that everyone knows what is meant, leaving some struggling to understand what it is that is being discussed. Definitions are therefore important right from the beginning of any attempt at integration.

Definitions of health seem to fall into two camps. One is where being healthy means a lack of illness or medically defined disease. The other implies that being healthy is connected to feelings of 'wellbeing', or the ownership of desired factors or qualities valued by society, such as weight and fitness. A general consensus followed the World Health Organization (WHO) statement which suggested that health was not merely an absence of disease or infirmity but 'a state of complete physical, mental and social wellbeing' (WHO, 1946), providing the bedrock of subsequent UK legislation. A further WHO publication *Learning Together to Work Together for Health* (WHO, 1988) encouraged diverse disciplines to come together to enhance knowledge and understanding.

When we talk of health care, we generally mean interventions that offer treatment or care for a specific medical condition, and it is the providers of these interventions who exert the greatest influence in assessing both needs and treatment. Traditionally, the strongest power base has resided in medicine (Freidson, 1970; Turner 1987), followed by nursing staff and other allied health professionals.

Definitions of social care are more complicated and we need to look at some of the legislation that has come into being since the 1960s to explore changing roles within social care. In terms of social work, following the Seebohm Committee Report (Seebohm, 1968) numerous children's services were brought under one umbrella. Shortly after, the Local Authority Social Services Act 1970 introduced new personal social services departments that integrated statutory social care and social provision within each local authority. These newly created departments covered all social problems 'from cradle to grave', and merged the role of individuals who had previously been members of distinct professions. Workers had seen themselves in a distinct 'pecking order', with those who had professionally qualified in their specialisation – psychiatric social workers, hospital almoners and child care officers – in first place, and welfare officers, who dealt mainly with elders and more generalised problems, coming last. The amalgamations of staff and equalising of pay were painful for many, who felt a loss of identity as well as professional title.

Social care has developed further since the publication of the Barclay Report (Barclay, 1982), advocating a community approach and the idea of partnerships within local communities to underpin the provision of social work. This report also argued that people could care more effectively for their own, and that social workers should support this. *The Children Act* (HMSO, 1989) and *Community Care Act* (HMSO, 1990) further altered structures so that the local authority and social work departments became purchasers of care rather than the main providers. The shift from direct provision to assessment of need, leading to purchase of 'care packages', opened the door to the private sector as a key social care provider. Later on in this chapter, policy regarding a combination of health and social care, and how it has influenced further change, will be discussed.

Policy, health, social care and integration

The case for integration of services lies in an economical use of resources, and more seamless packages of care. Better cohesion must surely result in efficient and relevant decision-making. However, the issue then arises of how to achieve integration without destroying professional identity. If integration is the desired goal, rather than assimilation, how do we retain ownership of what we are asked to do? It is also interesting, in this context, to ask who is responsible for health. Should individuals be responsible for their own health opportunities, or should health be seen as the responsibility of the state? Current health policy would appear to support the view that, while an individual's provision for private care is acceptable, the state should retain responsibility for the main provisions of health and social care. The contemporary imperative for current health and social care integration, however, derives from policy documents and circulars published in 2001 and 2002, mainly arising from legislation mentioned above. All reflect a change in social attitudes regarding health and wellbeing. Groups formed by patients, health authority committees and city partnerships have all served to bring into focus the importance of integrating services.

While the Health Act 1999 (HMSO, 1999) made it a statutory duty for the creation of partnerships between the NHS and local government, the primary legislation supporting changes in the NHS lies in the Health and Social Care Act 2001 (DoH, 2001a; Ch15, Sec11). The Act is intended to deliver aspects of *The NHS Plan* (DoH, 2000), but it is in the abundance of papers issued by the Department of Health that the issue of integration of services in health and social care is more fully addressed. For example, *The New NHS* (DoH, 1997) looks forward to the replacement of internal market forces by a 'system of integrated care, based on partnership and driven by performance'. *Our Healthier Nation: A Contract for Health* (DoH, 1998) cited, as causes of ill health, factors ranging from those beyond the individual to those determined by an individual. The same document also speaks of placing the duty on local authorities to work in partnerships with local people, local business and voluntary organisations. The *National Service Framework for Older People* (DoH, 2001b: 12) describes person-centred care being supported by 'newly integrated services'. Standard Two of the same document refers to the integrated provision of services. Perhaps the most telling introductions for integration lie in the formation of Health Improvement Programmes (HIPs) and Health Action Zones (HAZs).

HIPs were introduced in *The New NHS: modern, dependable* (DoH, 1997). These were then developed into Health Improvement and Modernisation Plans in *Saving Lives: Our Healthier Nation* (DoH, 1999a). They are expected to support the development of partnerships with local authorities, the voluntary sector and other organisations. These partnerships cover a wide spectrum of healthcare workers, social care workers, the voluntary sector, trades unions, schools, colleges and universities.

Established in April 1998, the HAZs are multi-agency partnerships, seen as 'trailblazers' in new ways of working and integrating services. Their purpose is to bring together local bodies relevant to health, with a view to agreeing strategies to improve local health. Reports on their progress are due in 2005 and will no doubt highlight what is being offered, and how it is being implemented. To date there is little informed comment on the process of gaining cooperation and coordination. There would appear to be an assumption, in policy statements and directives, that if a committee, group or partnership is formed from a variety of professional and lay representatives, then somehow integration of services will automatically follow. It is also worth considering that while this might be easier in city and large conurbations, it may not be so easy in the widespread rural areas. Anyone involved in healthcare and social care delivery is expected to assist in integrating the services so that 'seamless packages' of care are created. The quality of the interface between the two is crucial to this goal.

The health and social care interface

Historically, professions have set their own limits and produced codes of confidentiality and ethics. If the patient is now seen as central, professional identity should not be allowed to hinder integration of services to that patient. Not only the policy, but also the practice within health care and social care, needs to reflect this. It also follows that health and social care education should lead through the use of integrated methods of teaching and learning.

Collectively, patients seem to ask for better and more integrated care. The views of Expert Patient Groups established in 1999 (DoH, 1999b), the results of DoH Listening Exercises (Social Care Institute for Excellence [SCIE], 2002), plus input from the Patients Association to various governmental and local committees (The Patients Association, 2003), should add to the dialogue regarding the delivery of integrated care. Local Compacts (Home Office, 1998) looking at the interface between state and voluntary sectors may find that organisational politics need to be addressed if steering group memberships are to be 'even-handed'. Overall, integration of services seems the best way forward, and patients who are involved and engage in a supportive partnership with health and social care agents appear to respond in a positive way in terms of treatment outcomes (Salmon, 2000).

While medical staff may view professional autonomy as paramount, there may be less stress if decisions and responsibilities are shared more fully — especially in terms of the social aspects of patient care. The primary care initiative encourages multidisciplinary and inter-agency working, and it is to be hoped that different team members will take the lead at different times in terms of discussion and action. Medical practitioners are, however, used to exercising authority, and historically have had a great deal of autonomy. Social workers are also used to operating in this way, although other healthcare workers may not have traditionally taken the lead in care decisions (Bundred, 2001). Clearly, if integration of services is to occur, there has to be a change in the nature of the interface.

If integration is to be fully enacted, part of the way forward would seem to lie in education programmes. Most educators would agree that a better understanding of the roles and responsibilities of others produces more appropriate decision-making regarding both individual and general provisions (Rummery and Glendinning, 1997). Furthermore, if we are to think, primarily, of education and training as the way forward to achieving desired goals set out in policy, it is necessary to define the type of education desired and for whom it is intended.

Interprofessional education and training

IPE can be enacted at both pre- and post-qualification levels. The advantage of this lies in the argument that one needs to confirm one's own identity and practice before being confident enough to embrace those of another. Post-professional training allows for this. The drawback is that while the knowledge base about another's profession may be widened, individuals can retain inappropriate traditional ways of working, and associated prejudices. These issues need to be directly addressed within the post-qualification curriculum.

Multiprofessional education and training, sometimes called shared learning, involves joint sessions attended by representatives of all those professions involved. In terms of shared learning, however, along with content, the educational methods and baseline research need to be agreed. For example, research methods from social work (mainly qualitative), as opposed to those utilised in medical inquiry (mainly quantitative), require some accommodation and consensus that both are rigorous ways to collect and analyse data. The main advantage of multiprofessional collaborative learning would seem to lie in widening knowledge about the basic skills and practice of other professionals through shared approaches (Harden, 1998; Pirrie *et al*, 1998).

It might be suggested that we are inherently narcissistic, and will ask 'what's in it for me?' if well-tried and comfortable ways are to be changed or abandoned. Staff need to feel some sort of ownership of the ideas and proposed practice, and to appreciate that they hold more advantages than retaining the status quo. The aims, objectives and goals of proposed new ways of working, their effects on current practice, and how existing skills can still be used all need clarification. When government directives have been issued and change is required, rather than requested, the instigation of short courses is one way to help facilitate change in the workforce.

In brief, short courses can help staff to:

- manage the process of change where necessary
- build on current good practice
- identify 'what's in it for me', especially if 'old' methods are working for them
- create ownership of change.

Sustaining change is not easy, particularly if there are others in the working environment who object to new ways of working. Good practice learned can disappear like 'morning mist' unless it is nurtured. Confirmation of good practice through journal articles can help to sustain change. Refresher courses are also valuable, supported by more informal exchanges at local 'lunch groups'. The formation of a website specifically to exchange experiences and practical ideas is a useful information technology resource that can assist those who feel isolated or out of step. Exchange of teaching material, including interactive sites, can also be incorporated within the functions of the website.

Health and social care students who will operate integrative methods of practice are already in training, but the question of when and where training should be sited is still in discussion. Some think there is a need for the 'professional self' to be developed before engaging in multiprofessional dimensions of learning, while others think it should be earlier, so that unhelpful and entrenched attitudes are not learned, preventing the 'development of negative stereotypes' (Horder, 1996).

Two approaches to the timing of multidisciplinary education are:

- to deliver a common core followed by separate professional specialisation
- to use separate study modules in the promotion of a confident identity, followed by common modules.

Current medical student curriculum content that addresses integration at present appears to be sparse, apart from problem-based learning (PBL) groups and ad hoc provision of social care information or experience. Academic institutions, hospitals, GP practices or community-based organisations can host educational experiences, but the learning environment may influence content and how it is delivered. Methods are discussed elsewhere (Cooper *et al*, 2001), but experiential learning is already a part of some undergraduate medical courses, for example, those at Durham and Liverpool Universities.

Learning about others

It is now acknowledged that one important goal of IPE is to learn about the role of other professionals who contribute to the delivery of health care. One such initiative, at Liverpool University, has been to place second-year medical students outside the confines of hospital and primary settings, and into agencies that provide allied health or social care. Agencies vary from voluntary organisations that act as care providers for those with particular needs (learning difficulties, elderly, children with behaviour problems, etc) to organisations specifically formed to target vulnerable people (for example, victims of crime, drug and substance misusers, asylum seekers or ethnic groups). They may also be placed with healthcare personnel, such as community nurses or health visitors.

Their primary learning objective is to 'shadow' workers, experience how the service or organisation works and interfaces with other healthcare agencies, confirm determinants of health, and socially map the area within which they are placed. Project work is undertaken and a report of 2000 words has to embrace all the above issues, with an additional reflective section outlining what they have learned that they will be able to take with them in their future medical practice. An evaluation has been published (Cooper *et al*, 2001), which reveals an encouraging growth of understanding and skills in four key areas:

⌘ Multidisciplinary team working, intersectoral collaboration and an appreciation of the work and skills of other agencies, especially in the area of health care. Student's comments evidenced a wider awareness of the variety of needs that people have, and the array of resources to meet them. They also noted that they had changed their perceptions of the part that others play, especially in relation to assumptions about the central role of doctors in the care of patients. Stereotypes were challenged and students spoke of different perspectives on the stereotypical images they had grown up with.

⌘ The development of broader, humanistic, approaches to healthcare. Inequalities that effect the structuring of healthcare provision were highlighted alongside a better understanding of the complexities of the process of healthcare. Stronger feelings that health care really should be patient-centred were also expressed.

⌘ Increased interpersonal skills, particularly in terms of listening to patients and their carers, and a better understanding of non-verbal communication. The importance of accessibility to services was also noted.

⌘ A better understanding of the value of a community approach to health care, and awareness of the value of other services to healthcare beyond those relating to medicine.

Any type of community experience needs to make sense to students and other teaching staff. As more higher education institutions devise ways to include social care or community experiences in their medical curricula, it would be beneficial if methods and ideas could be exchanged, and a more uniform teaching/experiential learning process developed. If genuine multidisciplinary teaching occurs, students from nursing, allied professional health groupings and social workers could be taught together for particular modules. It should be remembered that many unpaid workers and carers exist in health and social care, and their experience should not be ignored.

Conclusion

There would appear to be a fair amount of agreement that, in addition to the skills necessary and desirable in the practice of their individual professions, we also want our future healthcare staff to learn about teamwork and collaboration (Walsh *et al*, 2000). These two attributes will include learning additional communication skills, understanding the parameters that constrain other professional workers, and appreciating the values that underpin their professional lives. All of these, along with knowledge of policies and structure in health and social care, will hopefully lead to better integration, as already envisaged in the rhetoric of assorted policy documents.

At the point of writing, integration of services is agreed regarding 'what' we want. The 'how' is still being developed, both in the management of change and in the education of future workers. While there is currently a great deal of debate regarding education of future workers, the management of change is not so readily discussed. The whole subject of health and social care integration is still in the melting pot. If integration is a reality – at least on paper – how this is measured in terms of patient satisfaction and seamless care is another matter. Hard evidence will need to come from practice regarding coordination, cooperation and decisions made regarding the packages of care to be delivered. No doubt, over the next few years we will see the evidence presented and be better able to decide whether integration is a reality in practice, or a myth created by policy writers.

References

Barclay PM (1982) *Social Workers: Their role and tasks*. National Institute for Social Work. Bedford Square Press, London.

Bundred P (2001) Health systems under pressure. In: Dowrick C (Ed). *Medicine in Society*. Arnold, London

Cooper H, Gibbs T, Brown L (2001) Community-oriented medical education. *Med Teach* **23**(3): 295–9

Department of Health (1990) *NHS and Community Care Act*. HMSO, London

Department of Health (1997) *The New NHS: Modern, dependable*. The Stationery Office, London

Department of Health (1998) *Our Healthier Nation: A contract for health*. The Stationery Office, London

Department of Health (1999a) *Saving Lives: Our healthier nation*. The Stationery Office, London

Department of Health (1999b) *The Expert Patient*. The Stationery Office, London

Department of Health (2000) *The NHS Plan. A plan for investment. A plan for reform*. The Stationery Office, London

Department of Health (2001a) *Health and Social Care Act*. The Stationery Office, London

Department of Health (2001b) *National Service Framework for Older People*. DoH, London

Fitzgerald M, Sim J (1982) *British Prisons*. Blackwell, Oxford

Freidson E (1970) *Profession of Medicine: A study of the sociology of applied knowledge*. New Dodd Mead, New York

Harden RM (1998) Multiprofessional education: part 1. *Med Teach* **20**(5): 402-8

HMSO (1989) *The Children Act*. The Stationery Office, London

HMSO (1999) *The Health Act*. The Stationery Office, London

Home Office (1998) *Compact: Getting it right together. Compact on relations between Government and voluntary and community sector in England* (Cm 4100). Home Office, London

Horder J (1996) The Centre for Advancement of Interprofessional Education. *Education for Health* **9**(3): 397-400

Patients Association (The) (2003) *Patient Voice* **18** and **19**. The Patients Association, London

Pirrie A, Wilson V, Harden, RM, Elsegood J (1998) Multiprofessional education: part 2. *Med Teach* **20**(5): 409–16

Rummery K, Glendinning C (1997) *Working Together: Primary care involvement in commissioning social care services*. Manchester National Primary Care Research & Development Centre, London

Salmon P (2000) *Psychology of Medicine and Surgery: A guide for psychologists, counsellors, nurses and doctors*. John Wiley, Chichester

Social Care Institute for Excellence (2002) *Listening Exercise Report*. SCIE, London

Seebohm F (1968) *Report of the Committee on Local Authority and Allied Personal Social Services*. HMSO, London

Turner BS (1987) *Medical Power and Social Knowledge*. Sage, London

Walsh M, Stephens P, Moore S (2000) *Social Policy and Welfare*. Stanley Thornes, Gloucester

World Health Organization (1946) *Constitution: Basic document*. WHO, Geneva

World Health Organization (1988) *Learning Together to Work Together for Health*. WHO, Geneva

4

Challenges facing the implementation of interprofessional education: a perspective from the allied health professions

Philip Turner

The term 'allied health professions' (AHPs) emerged with the publication of *Meeting the Challenge: A strategy for the allied health professions* (Department of Health [DoH], 2000a). This important policy document outlines their place in the modern National Health Service, establishing a clear set of strategic objectives encompassed within the following broad headings:

- contribution to modern care
- expanding the workforce
- modernising education, training and regulation
- career development
- making it happen.

The AHPs are a distinct group of professional staff, which include physiotherapists, speech and language therapists, occupational therapists and others who provide services that are essential in meeting the healthcare needs of patients and clients. This group are very diverse in their specialties. All are graduate-entry professions with the exception of paramedics. Some professions are not included, for example, clinical psychology, whose diagnostic and rehabilitative function might suggest that it should be included. One consistent feature linking the AHPs is that they are the first body of healthcare practitioners to be included, for registration purposes, within the Health Professions Council.

The diversity of these professional groupings suggests, however, that the application of a collective title alone is unlikely to ensure a collective approach to the future development of education and training. We need to consider how professional heterogeneity is organised and represented nationally within the NHS and higher education. Also, there is a need to explore how distinct occupational cultures have developed and how these might shape attitudes to issues such as interprofessional education (IPE).

The role of professional organisations

Each AHP has its own professional organisation, part of whose role involves defining, consolidating and developing the profession's identity and function. Membership of these professional organisations extends beyond the NHS workforce, and in some cases the majority of members are employed in the private sector.

Before publication of *Meeting the Challenge* (DoH, 2000a), the term 'professions allied to medicine' (PAMs) was loosely applied to an undefined collection of professions, who were neither medical nor nursing, but whose broad remit tended to be rehabilitative. Many professionals found this collective title misleading, primarily because it did not reflect the degree of clinical autonomy they exercised in clinical practice. The title also suggested a subordinate relationship to medical staff, and this did not enhance the kind of equitable relationships required for effective interdisciplinary team-working. It should be acknowledged, however, that the title PAM did reflect the relationship with medicine that existed in the infancy of many of these professional groups.

The professional organisations of the AHPs took a number of key steps towards redefining their roles and securing a more balanced relationship with other members of the healthcare team. These key developments are outlined in *Table 4.1*.

All of these activities have been made transparent by each professional organisation and are evidenced through their published business plans, strategies and annual reports. They are entirely in accord with their 'raison d'être' as guardians of standards, both for their members and for the users of their services. They also reflect the approaches taken by nursing and medical organisations.

The intention is that these changes will maximise the opportunities for each profession to influence the form and pace of change in the future. The identity of each profession has become aligned to the level and quality of its pre- and post-registration education and training, its standards of practice and the mechanisms in place to ensure and maintain the autonomy of its practitioners. The NHS modernisation agenda places an emphasis on the quality of service delivery and a growing involvement of service users in the development and monitoring of services. Any change to the structure and delivery of pre- and post-registration education, such as the introduction of IPE initiatives, must bear these issues in mind.

> ## Table 4.1: Changes led by the professional organisations
>
> ⌘ A growth in political awareness reflected in:
>
> - developed relationships with relevant user groups
> - increasingly sophisticated relationships with the media
> - increased investment in political lobbying
> - developed relationships with the Department of Health in order to inform and influence central strategy
>
> ⌘ The development of 'all-degree' pre-registration qualifications
>
> ⌘ The development of networks and post-registration training related to increasing specialisation within each discipline
>
> ⌘ The establishment and publication of minimum standards of practice for individuals and services and the subsequent development of professionally led audit, inspection or accreditation systems
>
> ⌘ The establishment of statutory or non-statutory professional registration systems – aligning practitioners to the published professional standards and, increasingly, requiring the provision of evidence of continuing professional development
>
> ⌘ The development of professional indemnity arrangements for members, reflecting the growth in clinical autonomy of each group

The Allied Health Professions Forum

Meeting the Challenge (DoH, 2000a) heralded the formation of the Allied Health Professions Forum as a key driver in implementation of the AHP strategy. The forum consists of both executive and elected officers from relevant professional bodies, with an elected chair. Despite its central role in realising the AHP strategy, it receives no apparent financial resources to support its function from the Department of Health.

The capacity of any individual professional body to effectively participate in the operation and development of the forum is dependent upon both its relative size and disposition to engage. Half of the forum's members, including the chair, are elected officers with limited tenures. This presents a considerable challenge in terms of consistency and continuity. This, combined with the likelihood of divergent objectives and specific interests of member organisations, make it an unlikely driver of the substantial change envisaged within the *NHS Plan* (DoH, 2000b), including recommendations around IPE.

The organisation of AHPs in the NHS and other healthcare organisations

'Shifting the Balance of Power' is the programme of change brought about to empower frontline staff and patients in the NHS. The main documents published as part of this programme have defined new organisational structures and responsibilities (DoH, 2001, 2002). As well as clarifying the role of primary care trusts, the programme sets out the responsibilities of strategic health authorities and the directorates of health and social care. It does not, however, specify how AHPs might relate effectively to these new structures, or participate in the process of modernisation and strategic development. The matter was confused further for AHPs when the NHS announced the dissolution of the directorates of health and social care in January 2003.

There are wide variations across the country in the structuring of AHPs, both within and across health and social care boundaries. Typically, these professional groups are likely to be employed by a range of local organisations providing health and social care to individual healthcare providers. Historically, AHPs have endeavoured, often unsuccessfully, to aggregate into larger groupings, in an attempt to develop a critical mass and exert influence upon their parent organisations. Conversely, NHS trusts have reorganised services into functional directorates, such as surgery or medicine.

Professional groups within NHS trusts are, typically, organised and managed at directorate level. Although it has not been formally evaluated, the capacity of AHPs to influence local strategy and become involved in the process of modernisation is, at best, variable. While the strategic capacity of AHPs is markedly compromised, their diversity and distribution provide them with the potential to be influential in the process of NHS modernisation.

At a service delivery level, AHPs work within clinical teams, often operating at the interface between organisations and external agencies. Management arrangements for staff in these teams are often complex. Effective team-working, though, requires interdisciplinary working practices to overcome both professional and organisational divisions. It is likely that these environments provide some of the most fertile ground for the development of an interdisciplinary culture.

Examples would include:

⌘ Intermediate care services combining a range of nursing and social care disciplines across primary care, acute and social services boundaries.

⌘ Services to children with special needs, bringing together educationalists, speech and language therapists and other rehabilitation disciplines.

Where team-working breaks down, the stated reason is often that of perceived territorial incursion beyond an acceptable point. The injured party's concerns often revolve around a perception that another team member is operating outside of acknowledged boundaries, in a manner that presents risks to the patient or the professional integrity of the team member. Such conflicts can stifle innovation and mutual understanding.

The NHS Plan (DoH, 2000b) and *Meeting the Challenge* (DoH, 2000a) introduced significant changes to the organisational culture of the NHS and its partner organisations. Necessarily, education and training for health workers represents one element of culture change, with the intent to provide a broader skills base and a more integrated approach to the delivery of care.

Change management strategies will be a critical factor in determining the extent to which workforce members become involved in the process of planning, shaping and implementing change. If NHS structures do not enable the effective engagement of the AHP workforce, in an equal partnership with other colleagues, then the implementation of change is likely to be more difficult for all concerned.

Key strategic objectives for the AHPs

There are more than 50,000 allied health professionals working in the NHS in England, representing 7–8% of the clinical workforce, compared with nursing, which constitutes 69%. The publication of *Meeting the Challenge* (DoH, 2000a) represents the first occasion when the important contribution of the AHPs has been acknowledged by the Department of Health in a strategic document. New regulatory arrangements bringing together all AHPs, through the establishment of the Health Professions Council, have the potential to support interprofessional working through the development of explicit guidelines on IPE. This document also indicates a number of key areas where IPE is likely to make a significant contribution towards achieving the strategy.

Allied health professionals work within priority areas such as cancer, diabetes and older people. Many work across agency boundaries and are therefore likely to be key professionals in decision-making related to schemes that give health and local authorities the capacity to pool budgets and develop increasingly integrated services. These priority areas might logically reflect the most appropriate areas within which to explore models of IPE at both pre- and post-registration level, not least because of the increased likelihood of funding support.

Meeting the Challenge (DoH, 2000a) reported future investment in the form of additional resources to strengthen the link between continuing professional development (CPD) and registration. It also announced the intention to establish a new career and grading structure with the capacity to reflect the increased flexibility required within the roles and responsibilities of staff working in integrated teams. This included the introduction of a therapist consultant grade, with the intention of encouraging the wider involvement of allied health professionals in high-level clinical leadership. The increasing flexibility offered by new career and salary structures provides opportunities to create posts that can cross traditional professional boundaries. This need not be purely at a clinical level, but could also involve the development of professional education posts, possibly as joint posts with the higher education institutions (HEIs), the remit of which could incorporate IPE. Specifically mentioned are the development of common foundation programmes, flexible pathways into and through pre-registration programmes, and joint training in core skills.

The AHP strategy admirably sets the scene for the development of IPE, in terms of its statements of strategic intent, its allocation of resources and its development of conditions to encourage the development of interprofessional roles and relationships between higher education and service providers. The strategy is less clear about how, specifically, AHPs will be better enabled to influence the strategic agenda. While the 'Shifting the Balance of Power' programme defines a number of responsibilities for the now defunct directorate of health and social care and strategic health authorities, there is no indication of how, structurally, these might be met. This may be because the AHP strategy was released at a time of major organisational change in the NHS. It might also reflect the fact that AHPs have, in general, not been afforded any representative or inclusive structures beyond local level in the past, and it has not yet been thought important that they should in the future.

The development of interprofessional education

In the past, each professional body had the legislated responsibility for accrediting its own pre-registration education. This provided the vehicle for the establishment of 'all-degree' professions. This role is now undertaken by the newly established Health Professions Council the Joint Validation Committee, comprising representatives from each professional body. Thus, the regulation of AHPs is within the remit of a single organisation. This provides greater opportunity to explore professional overlap and reflect this within accreditation requirements.

Obstacles to the development of IPE at pre-registration level, however, are more to do with uncertainties about the process of change than the inherent attitude of the professions. HEIs must satisfy accreditation requirements in order to maintain the viability of pre-registration provision. The main initiators of change in the nature and content of curricula was originally informed by the Workforce Development Conferations. These have now been replaced by the Strategic Health Authorities (SHAs). On behalf of their constituent trusts and health authorities, the SHAs develop contracts with local HEIs determining student numbers and course content. It is conceivable that changes required by SHAs may be incompatible with the requirements of the Joint Validation Committee. This places HEIs in the unenviable position of having to satisfy 'two masters', one with the money and one with the legislative authority.

If accreditation obstacles can be overcome, there are a number of practical difficulties arising from the relative size and distribution of courses within and among HEIs. The early development of integrated pre-registration education is likely to take place across a range of different disciplinary combinations and may be more likely to focus on the integration of various AHP groupings, than the integration of AHPs with nursing or medicine. This is primarily due to a disproportionate ratio of student numbers across the professions. For example, nursing intakes are often in cohorts of hundreds compared with below 70 for AHPs. Additionally, nursing recruits more than one intake of students per year, leading to conflict in terms of timing of academic and clinical content to accommodate IPE. Initiatives focused on the development of the post-registration and assistant workforce are likely to be easier to implement.

Typically, AHPs work in teams with each other and other health and social care disciplines. Most teams have developed a supporting workforce of assistant grade staff, and these increasingly fulfil a role that straddles the boundaries of a number of professions. For example, rehabilitation assistants may work in supportive roles in occupational therapy, physiotherapy, speech and language therapy, social care and nursing. Likewise, classroom assistants support the work of teachers and other therapists in education. The National Vocational Qualifications (NVQ) framework accredits the skills and competencies of this staff group.

There must be room to further develop interprofessional working through more structured IPE. Much of this training and development can take place in the workplace and be delivered by professional colleagues with supervisory responsibilities. The requirement to train and develop their assistant staff in an integrated manner is likely to also develop more integrated thinking and practice among qualified team members. We should also use the skills of experienced assistants to support the training of pre- and post-registration health professionals. Established multiprofessional teams provide an ideal environment for the implementation of post-registration IPE. Local initiatives will remain fragmented and uncoordinated unless SHAs and clinical networks become constructively involved.

It would be helpful if the SHAs' workforce plans incorporated the following actions:

- to develop an overview of local initiatives, generating and supporting new ideas
- to disseminate new and good practice among their partner organisations and other confederations
- to promote partnership arrangements with higher education and the Health Professions Council.

In conclusion, the current environment offers opportunities to develop IPE that will greatly enhance the interprofessional delivery of health and social care. Partnerships between professional groupings and statutory bodies are crucial to the realisation of the IPE vision. There are some cultural and structural obstacles that need to be acknowledged before they can be overcome.

References

Department of Health (2000a) *Meeting the Challenge: A strategy for the allied health professions.* DoH, London

Department of Health (2000b) *The NHS Plan. A plan for investment. A plan for reform.*
DoH, London

Department of Health (2001) *Securing Delivery.* DoH, London

Department of Health (2002) *Next Steps.* DoH, London

5

Interprofessional learning: curriculum development, approval and delivery in higher education

Marilyn Hammick

This chapter discusses issues that arise in higher education (HE) curriculum planning, development, approval and delivery, where interprofessional learning is part of health and social care courses that lead to both academic and professional awards. The major emphasis is on the development of interprofessional education (IPE) since getting this right minimises the challenges associated with gaining approval and implementing the programme. Aspects discussed include preparation, staffing, and curriculum characteristics. Before moving to these substantive topics, I want to make brief reference to two semantic issues.

The chapter title uses the term approval, for which I could have substituted accreditation, validation and endorsement; the list is not exhaustive. The use of one particular word is frequently part of a particular professional tradition. This is an example of the language conflicts that can easily arise in interprofessional work. For simplicity, I use the term 'approval' to embrace all those processes that confer formal, official recognition of worthiness, or a kite mark, by a professional, statutory or academic body. Issues related to seeking joint academic and professional approval are discussed later.

The focus in this chapter is mainly on curricula that are explicitly interprofessional. It is also useful to remember that IPE may be integrated or implicit within curricula for health and social care awards where practitioners from different professions learn together. This multiprofessional learning, which is also referred to as common learning or shared learning, does not necessarily promote collaborative practice. However, IPE may also be referred to as shared, common or multiprofessional learning, and there are other definitions and terms also used to describe such courses.

Here, I am discussing IPE that is designed to promote collaboration, and which uses interactive learning methods to do this. As defined, IPE can be the explicit purpose of a short course, an explicit and discrete part of the curriculum of a long, award-bearing course, or integrated throughout the curriculum of a longer course. Deciding which of these models of IPE you are involved in is essential. It will enable course development to focus on issues of relevance and will signify conceptual clarity about the curriculum design to the approval panel.

The majority of IPE involving practitioners from the allied health professions and nursing takes place after initial professional qualification, and is almost always within service settings (Freeth *et al*, 2002). In contrast, pre-qualifying interprofessional learning more usually takes place either in HE settings or as part of a practice attachment. Early agreement about the location of the education event is essential. This is especially important where resources may need to be enhanced to accommodate the planned learning activity.

Learning to collaborate can also take place within multiprofessional courses. Learning may be organised to realise the potential for this or it may be the unplanned result of practitioners simply learning together. Additionally, for most long award-bearing professional courses, the importance of learning about interprofessional team-work during practice attachments cannot be underestimated. Again, this may not be explicitly stated within, for example, the learning outcomes of the clinical education curriculum.

Although this is less than ideal, within certain political and professional contexts, it may be all that can be hoped for. In these curricula, given present policy initiatives to prepare all health and social care practitioners for collaborative work, the overall course aims may hint at enabling successful students to participate in collaborative work practices. Indeed, it is difficult to see where approval would be given were this not so, given current political imperatives to encourage teamwork and inter-agency cooperation (Secretary of State for Health, 2000). In these situations, it is helpful to reflect these policies, in some way, within the curriculum, and to adopt some of the practices suggested below to enhance the potential for students to learn to work interprofessionally.

Course development, approval and delivery: joined-up processes

If you are involved in developing, seeking, giving approval or delivering courses that are interprofessional in any of the above ways, you will need to focus on the key issues, discussed below, that characterise interprofessional aspects of the pedagogy. For clarity and convenience, these processes (development, approval and delivery) are often referred to separately. This recognises that they occupy discrete time periods in the life of a course and that there are some unique aspects to each process. However, experience indicates that, in practice, there is not necessarily, or even ideally, a distinction between them.

One of the essential aspects of developing, gaining approval and delivering a successful course is continuity and collaboration between all those involved. The need for a 'joined-up' approach from the time when the ideas for any course are discussed, and throughout all its subsequent development and delivery, is arguably even more important with interprofessional and multiprofessional education. Another reason for smoothing the divisions between the three processes lies in the very nature of the work itself. Education is a human and social process, and professional practice learning is subject to an ever-changing context. Health and social care curricula need to respond to policy changes if future practitioners are to be equipped to practise in the real world of their patients and clients. Nowhere is this more so than in the interprofessional arena, where there is an increasing emphasis on collaborative working and emerging evidence for the effectiveness of IPE across a wide range of different educational settings (Secretary of State for Health, 2000; Freeth *et al*, 2002).

Ideally, development, approval and delivery are integrated parts of an iterative process that seeks to engage with current issues in the field. In this model, development is evolutionary and continuous; approval recognises the need for some flexibility in the curriculum, and delivery involves being alert to new policies and practices on behalf of the students.

Development, approval and delivery: preparation and timelines

The process of course planning should begin with a clear and shared understanding of how long development and approval may take, who is likely to be involved, and the location of all this activity. Time spent on planning all three processes will ensure that the development team are aware of the time they will need to commit to the processes, where and when meetings will be held, and how the team will function in respect of producing the documentation normally required by, first, the approving bodies, and then the students and staff delivering the education.

The timeline for the development will vary considerably depending on whether you are developing a short course in response to a local need or planning a three-year undergraduate course leading to co-terminus awards of an honours degree and a professional registration to practise. *Table 5.1* summarises the timelines for both types of courses.

Table 5.1: Key timelines for short and long courses		
Process	**Short course**	**Long course**
Development	Days to months	Months to years
Approval	Brief: but may be dependent on the administrative procedures of another organisation	Months and may be dependent on the administrative procedures of multiple organisations
Delivery	Days to weeks	Years

Recent systematic reviews of the effectiveness of IPE have revealed a wide range of different practitioners learning together and doing so at all times during their career (Freeth *et al*, 2002; Hammick *et al*, 2002). One feature that these courses have in common with other types of education is that the quality of the final outcome is dependent upon having the right team of people working effectively together, with commitment to the task and sufficient time to do the work involved. This is even more important for the development, approval and delivery of IPE and can be much more difficult to achieve. The next section outlines the reasons for this and suggests ways of achieving effective collaboration within the course team.

Staff issues

The staff involved in course planning and approval will need to reflect the aims of the interprofessional learning they are designed to facilitate: working collaboratively, as a team, with respect for colleagues. Achieving this requires patience, good planning and a well-developed sense of professionalism. The team leader will need interpersonal skills of the highest order to enable members with diverse professional and educational backgrounds to have the confidence to make their unique contribution to the curriculum, and the courage to leave other aspects of their 'baggage' for another time. Team members may be on different sites, from different universities, and bring diverse experiences of course development and approval events.

As *Table 5.2* indicates, for short courses there may be a ready-made planning team, motivated to produce a training course to meet a specific service need and used to working together. Even so, their familiarity with each other may be as clinical colleagues, working alongside but at a distance, perhaps only communicating through patients' notes, referral letters or brief meetings focused on a clinical problem. They may not (yet) have the skills necessary for membership of a team that can effectively develop and deliver IPE.

Planning a long award course will involve a large number of staff, from different professions, working in academic and clinical settings. These teams may also take time to adjust to the border crossing necessary in interprofessional work. Teams like this will inevitably pass through the stages of team-making, able to perform only after they have got to know each other (formed), ironed out potential conflicts (stormed) and accepted the interprofessional norms of the team (Palmer, 1988). Allowing time for team-making will enhance the success of the work done. For short courses, this process may have to happen quickly.

For a team that aims to plan and deliver a full-time undergraduate course with discrete interprofessional modules, working closely together for several months, the team-making process may not necessarily be linear. At critical times, for example, following an internal approval event that results in further and demanding work on the curriculum, team life may be stormy and re-norming may need to take place. The course development team may also need to overcome the management pressures on staff. Representing an organisation where policy directives seek decreased costs through shared learning opportunities can be stressful during the development of education that requires a joined-up and interactive approach to learning.

Table 5.2: Key features of staffing for short and long courses		
Process	**Short course**	**Long course**
Development	Team motivated by patient/client/service focused needs	Predetermined, large faculty team of old and new colleagues, together with practitioners from diverse settings
Approval	Peer review Internal, informal External, brief documentation	Peers from other universities and nominated by professional and stautory bodies
Delivery	Development team ± limited external speakers or trainers	Faculty and practitioners

Table 5.3 shows some of the key features that the clinical and educational staff developing the course will need to share. A successful interprofessional curriculum for students from different professions will be dependent upon each recognising the others' contributions to clinical care, alternative theoretical paradigms and possibilities for new learning and teaching methods. The interprofessional course development team will need to manage curriculum pressures arising from balancing learning about appropriate models of care and learning about how to deliver that care as a team.

Ideally, the planning team will also include student and service user representatives. The importance of members who can offer these different perspectives on education is undeniable.

Table 5.3: Key features that clinical and educational staff developing the course will need to share
❖ Values
❖ Ethics
❖ Reciprocity
❖ Mutual respect
❖ Collaborative working
❖ Common learning
❖ Comparative learning
❖ Interprofessional assessment
❖ Joint learning outcomes

The added value of their contribution is, however, at the potential price of additional tensions, as even more diverse opinions are available to shape the curriculum. It can also be difficult for students to find the time to get to meetings. Alternative ways of seeking their views, for example, taking specific questions to a student group meeting or asking for written comments on draft papers, often need to be found.

Individual team members representing one particular perspective on care can feel weighted down by their responsibility. This is more likely to happen if they are the only members of their particular group and if, traditionally, their views have been given less credence in education planning. This is similar to how the single profession student can feel as part of an interprofessional seminar or problem-based learning group. In this way, experiencing the process of course development mirrors the educational experience for the students. A course development team that can reflect on their experiences can usefully shape the interprofessional curriculum with this in mind.

Key features

Interprofessional curriculum development

It is the process of developing an IPE curriculum that determines the outcome of the approval and delivery stages. This is probably why course development can feel painful, takes time, and shares characteristics with the process of education it seeks to develop. The interprofessional curriculum needs to be developed with care, for example, giving attention to language, culture, and the complementary and unique nature of each student's knowledge and skills, and recognising the different experiences they each bring. Particularly for courses leading to academic and professional awards there is a need to be aware of the potential for conflicts in the achievement of learning outcomes that support professional autonomy and those that focus on collaborative working. Consideration of these underlying aspects of the curriculum, in relation to both the course content and the education process, has greater potential to facilitate learning how to work interprofessionally, without a constructed boundary around the group and with transparent borders between them.

Interprofessional approval

Approval of an educational event differs according to features such as the type of course, its intention and length. Almost always, the process involves some form of peer review and requires documentary evidence about the curriculum. Formal approval of educational programmes for health and social care practitioners is always sought for long courses leading to a qualification that signifies that the successful student is competent to practise his or her profession. Universities validate courses to ensure that they comply with university regulations and to demonstrate consistency across courses. Professional and statutory bodies confer accreditation in recognition that a programme provides some, or all, of the competencies needed for professional practice. These two processes aim to ensure fitness for award and fitness for practice respectively. While they seek to be harmonious, a course team trying to meet their individual requirements is often faced with considerable challenges. Awarding bodies have customs and practices that may not harmonise with those of their partners in the approval process. It is useful for the course development team to have some insight into the awarding bodies' working ways at approval events. Asking questions of colleagues with this experience is one way of being prepared for the idiosyncrasies of panel members from particular organisations.

For most university-based courses that also lead to a practice qualification the professional and statutory bodies' requirement is for the awards to be co-terminus: in other words, the professional and academic awards must be given at the same time and one will not be given without the other. Where students exit a course without the professional qualification, it is usually with a differently named award from the one that is co-terminus with professional registration. During the development of the course it is useful to plan for this possibility and seek approval of this non-registrable award. This forward thinking can alleviate the problems that may ensue when it becomes clear that students will not be eligible for the professional practice award but are entitled to recognition of their academic achievements.

Short IPE courses, such as a clinical audit workshop, may be considered a continuing professional development (CPD) event by the participants. Recent legislative changes in the UK mean that health and social care practitioners must produce evidence of their CPD. For nurses and midwives this means meeting the requirements of the Post-registration and Practice (PREP) CPD standard of a minimum thirty-five hours' learning activity over three years. For practitioners regulated by the new Health Professions Council, registration will be linked with evidence of CPD. This will have an impact on all manner of CPD provision, including IPE, with an expansion in the need to seek accreditation of short courses from professional and registration bodies. Educational initiatives that previously may have not been thought of as CPD may increasingly need to include evidence of accreditation. For example, quality improvement initiatives and clinical audit workshops, with their focus on guideline development or improvement, are often interprofessional in nature. For examples see Spencer *et al* (1993) and Hunter and Love (1996).

Professional bodies vary in their approaches to this, and for many it is a simple and speedy process. The Royal College of Physicians, for example, offers information on the process and the necessary forms on its website (www.rcplondon.ac.uk). A number of professional organisations, such as The General Dental Council, are now asking for verifiable CPD. This means supplying evidence of full participation in the CPD and, in some cases, proof of achievement of the learning outcomes. Staff organising short courses need to take these developments into account in the early phases of course development.

Planning and preparation is the key to successful accreditation, and nowhere is this more necessary than for the complex and challenging validation events that are often associated with the academic and professional approval of interprofessional learning for two or more health and social care practitioner groups. Pilot events, informal peer review of documents, and a team that owns and believes in the course it is presenting will all minimise the anxieties that both the internal and external approval events can cause. An important aspect of course development is the support from senior faculty staff to the development team. This includes providing evidence that the partnerships between education and service settings to deliver the IPE are based on realistic resource agreements, and clearly indicate roles and responsibilities of the staff involved.

Members of approval panels also have a responsibility to ensure that the approval process is another example of collaborative working and not a confrontational and negative encounter. Experience and expertise in IPE varies across institutions and professions. *Benchmarking Academic and Practitioner Standards in Health Care Subjects, Medicine* (Quality Assurance Agency, 2001, 2002) etc. are only of minimal guidance in respect of competence and capability in collaborative working. Evidence of effectiveness of IPE is increasing, but there are still gaps in our knowledge about what works for different professional groups, and in what circumstances.

All this indicates an underdeveloped pedagogy, where creative approaches to course design and delivery are welcome (as long as there are plans to evaluate their effectiveness) and diverse approaches to achieving interprofessional learning outcomes are to be expected. In this situation, as long as the course development team are able to argue their case, it behoves the approving bodies to accept diversity in interprofessional curricula.

Delivering interprofessional education

Finally, a brief look at issues that may arise following course approval – just when you might think that all the challenges are behind you. Putting an interprofessional curriculum into practice brings resource, organisational and administrative challenges that can have a lasting and less than positive influence on staff and student views of learning together to work together. *Table 5.4* shows a selection of the issues that need attention to ensure that IPE is delivered satisfactorily.

The list of issues given in *Table 5.4* is not exhaustive. They vary depending

Table 5.4: Challenges associated with delivering interprofessional education

Resources
* Teaching staff
* Staff training
* Staff development
* External examiners

Organisation
* Location of teaching
* Size and number of teaching rooms
* Coincidental teaching appointments
* External examiners

Administration
* Support staff
* Timetabling
* Exam boards
* Student recruitment

on the length of the course or module and existing facilities. Difficulties may especially arise with large cohorts of students, when course participants are located at different sites and when teaching staff are inadequately prepared for interprofessional pedagogy.

Conclusion

The outline of the work required to develop, gain approval and deliver IPE given in this chapter has, by necessity, left much unwritten. It has focused on general issues, which are of potential value to staff involved in these processes for any type of education, including CPD and long award courses. The key points elaborated in the chapter are summarised below. Essentially these provide a foundation that will enhance the experiences of developing, approving, and delivering IPE for staff, and, importantly, will assist in providing students with an optimal learning experience.

KEY POINTS

⌘ Decide and document the model of interprofessional education (IPE) you are working with and the location of the planned education event.

⌘ Planning timelines for the development, approval and delivery processes is an important early task.

⌘ Staff involved in the planning and approval of IPE will need to work collaboratively, as a team, and with respect for their colleagues.

⌘ Interprofessional curricula require care and attention during their development, given the potential for professional conflicts inherited from the more traditional forms of health and social care education.

⌘ Approval is a peer review process; its form depends on course length, but it is increasingly unusual not to seek some type of official kite mark for an education event.

⌘ Delivering an interprofessional course has resource, organisational and administrative implications.

References

Freeth D, Hammick M, Koppel I, Reeves S, Barr H (2002) *A Critical Review of Evaluations of Interprofessional Education*. Learning and Teaching Support Network Health Sciences and Practice, London

Hammick M, Barr H, Freeth D, Koppel I, Reeves S (2002) Systematic reviews of evaluations of IPE: results and work in progress. *J Interprof Care* **16**(1): 80–4

Hunter M, Love C (1996) Total Quality Management and the reduction of inpatient violence and cost in a forensic psychiatric hospital. *Psychiatr Serv* **47**(75): 1–54

Palmer JD (1988) For the manager who must build a team. In: Reddy WB, Jamison K (Eds). *Team Building*. Institute for Applied Behavioral Science, Virginia, and University Associates, Inc, San Diego, California: 137–49

Quality Assurance Agency for Higher Education (2001) *Benchmarking Academic and Practitioner Standards in Health Care Subjects/Professions*. Quality Assurance Agency for Higher Education, Gloucester

Quality Assurance Agency for Higher Education (2002) *Benchmarking Standards in Medicine*. Quality Assurance Agency for Higher Education, Gloucester

Secretary of State for Health (2000) *The NHS Plan*. Department of Health, London

Spencer J, Pearson P, James P, Southern A (1993) *Improving the Way we Work: Report of a multidisciplinary audit project*. University of Newcastle upon Tyne, Newcastle

Part 2

Planning, Implementing and Evaluating Interprofessional Education in Practice

6

Communication skills training in cancer care using actors as simulated patients

Tom Donovan, Dave Mercer and Ray Sutton

Communication skills training in cancer care settings is a priority area for improvement and development within current healthcare policy. Using a multiprofessional communication skills programme, and drawing upon the experience of educationalists and actors, this chapter explores a challenging topic that is currently the subject of widespread debate.

Communication in cancer care

Despite marked improvements in its management and prognosis, a diagnosis of cancer remains a distressing and worrying event. In addition to the physical and social disruption engendered through the illness and its treatment, many people with cancer experience considerable psychological, emotional or psychiatric disruption at some point following diagnosis (Derogatis *et al*, 1983). Effective communication is a crucial element in the accurate assessment of patient concerns and the subsequent provision of psychosocial support. Conversely, inadequate or ineffective communication can be the basis of considerable distress for patients and compromise psychological adjustment to the cancer diagnosis (Kruijver *et al*, 2000). However, for many health professionals, talking to patients about these emotional and psychological issues is a source of considerable distress. Issues such as diagnosis, prognosis and terminal illness present significant challenges to health professionals, who frequently feel ill prepared to deal with the 'difficult' questions that such conversations generate. Lack of training, fear of saying the 'wrong thing' or 'making matters worse' are frequently cited by health professionals as reasons for avoiding these 'difficult conversations' (Wilkinson, 1991; Heaven and Maguire, 1996).

Several studies suggest that some health professionals intuitively adopt a range of strategies designed to 'ease' the communication process. These 'blocking behaviours' (Maguire *et al*, 1996) are often used to minimise the discomfort of health professionals rather than addressing patient needs. Typical blocking behaviours include:

Selective attention: This occurs when health professionals control the content of a conversation to avoid discussing 'difficult' emotional issues. For example:

Patient: *I've had this pain recently and I'm terrified that the cancer might be coming back.*

Nurse: *Tell me about this pain, is it worse at night?*

Switching focus: 'Switching' can occur in several contexts. Health professionals may switch topics, time frame or person focus to steer conversations into less challenging areas. For example:

Patient: *Thinking about this illness makes me feel so frightened.*

Nurse: *So how is your wife coping with things?*

Passing the buck:

Patient: *I'm worried about what this will mean for my family and me.*

Nurse: *In that case, I'll refer you to the Macmillan nurse.*

Unfortunately, several of these widely used tactics result in confusion, misunderstanding, unrealistic prognoses and, at worst, complete breakdown in the patient- professional relationship. Central health policy documents (Department of Health [DoH], 1995, 2000) acknowledge the urgent need to address the issue, and plans are underway to find the most effective ways of improving both clinical outcomes and patient experience. Given that effective communication is an essential element in the roles of many of the health professionals who work with cancer patients, it would appear that interprofessional training in this area is a logical extension of educational provision.

Breaking down barriers to communication

A key issue in preparing health professionals to deal effectively with the challenges of communicating with cancer patients resides in their educational preparation. Until the past few decades, communication skills were rarely included in pre-qualification education, and specific communication issues relating to cancer care were usually found within the exclusive domain of psycho-oncology. Fortunately, through a range of educational initiatives within the NHS and the independent hospice sector, this situation has markedly improved.

The key to breaking down barriers to communication lies in the recognition that health professionals and patients frequently have separate and, often, competing agendas. Communication breaks down or becomes ineffective when the patient's agenda is subsumed by the health professional's priorities. Within a multiprofessional context, these issues become further complicated and enmeshed, as role-specific aims and outcomes compete for precedence within multiprofessional teams. In typical multi-disciplinary teams in cancer settings, the range of health professionals involved could encompass oncologists, surgeons, pathologists, nurses, dietitians and physiotherapists. Thus the communication skills required for such a team could range from simple information-giving to breaking 'bad news', or initiating therapeutic interventions. *Table 6.1* illustrates just a few of the important issues that different health professionals may have to address in relation to communication in cancer settings.

Table 6.1: Examples of multiprofessional learning priorities	
Dietitians	Information giving, accurate nutritional assessment, changing prior eating behaviour, coping with diminished appetite
Doctors	Diagnosis disclosure, prognosis disclosure, explaining treatments, breaking bad news
Radiographers	Simplifying complex information, answering 'difficult' questions, explaining side-effects
Nurses	Therapeutic psychological interventions, supportive care after bad news, psychosocial support, communicating with relatives

The challenge, for the interprofessional education (IPE) facilitator, is to design a learning experience that provides skills to ultimately enhance communication and support for cancer patients, and address the diverse range and levels of communication involved in contemporary multiprofessional practice. Although individual health professionals must learn the requisite skills for their own practice, IPE offers the opportunity, within the context of communication, for practitioners to understand how their roles complement each other, and how best to use this in a shared way to enhance care provision.

The next section discusses some pragmatic issues arising from the experience of an 'in-service' multiprofessional communication skills course within a large NHS trust. The programme was delivered over two days, and was offered, free of charge, to nurses and allied health professionals.

Communication skills training in healthcare settings should provide students with opportunities to develop skills, explore their own feelings and attitudes, and identify the extent of their learning needs. However, initiating and developing in-service learning opportunities frequently presents difficulties to programme facilitators. The reality of providing effective healthcare in the NHS requires skilled and experienced personnel, able to deliver complex and demanding care interventions twenty-four hours a day. Consequently, health professionals invariably find little available time for continuing education. Where learning opportunities exist, the drive to develop 'new ways of working' (DoH, 1999) and breaking down traditional uniprofessional role boundaries means that health professionals must judiciously select those learning opportunities that afford the most valuable 'returns', offer value for money, and correspond with the time demands of contemporary practice. Implicitly, a key feature of the learning experience must be its relevance and application to practice.

Background and aims

Imposing a set of broad aims on any educational experience helps facilitators to crystallise learning outcomes, and is invaluable in shaping the programme to meet the outcome requirements (Reece and Walker, 1997). However, unless the aims and outcomes are shared and 'owned' by the learners, the programme will primarily serve the agenda of the programme provider. A unidirectional approach could disadvantage learners, where aspects of the learning programme have little relevance to their practice. This issue is further complicated in multiprofessional learning arenas where priorities for different elements of the programme vary among participants. One approach to this is to set general learning outcomes and invite students to develop their own learning agenda (Wilkinson *et al*, 1999). This approach confers advantages by identifying individual learning needs, and allows programme facilitators and learners to reach a consensus on the topics and issues to be covered during the learning experience.

Table 6.2 presents examples of some broad aims and student-generated topics. When students identify specific problems from practice, role-play is used as a means of trying out alternative approaches to evaluate the effectiveness of each. Every student then has an opportunity, throughout the programme, to 'try out' different elements of the scenario. For example, one student might begin the role-play to focus upon opening a dialogue, another might deal with difficult questions and another could attempt problem-solving with the 'patient'. In this way, students acquire new skills and, in the context of IPE, develop an appreciation of how other roles are sometimes more appropriate to deal with common problems. For example, one course participant (a nurse) commented:

> *'I never thought of asking a dietitian for help when my patient's appetite was poor. I used to just give them milky drinks. I didn't realise that there were other things that we could do.'*

Table 6.2: Broad learning aims and student-generated topics	
Broad aims of the programme (general)	❖ To provide an opportunity for students to share common experiences and challenges in communication ❖ To review theoretical issues relating to the psychological care of an individual with cancer ❖ To enhance existing communication skills ❖ To develop new communication skills to aid assessment and support
Student-generated topics (specific)	Patient education; worries about eating; coping with reduced mobility; diagnosis disclosure; prognosis disclosure, explaining treatments; 'breaking bad news'; 'picking up the pieces'; managing collusive relationships; dealing with anger; identifying depressed patients; supporting relatives

Structure and style

A primarily student-led agenda provides fewer opportunities for teachers to prioritise the topics that students 'must' know in order to understand theoretical issues and contextualise the learning experience. A didactic theoretical element can invite shared viewpoints and role-specific contributions from participants. While theoretical issues contextualise the topic and provide meaningful insights, the key element of this form of educational experience is the experiential 'hands-on' approach to learning. The programme illustrated in *Table 6.3* shows a typical programme containing student-generated themes and facilitator-led theoretical elements. This type of programme is appropriate for a cohort of around ten to twelve participants.

Table 6.3: A typical programme

Time	Topic	Teaching and learning mode
DAY 1		
09.00	Introduction	
09.15	Agenda setting: • What problems do *you* experience when communicating with cancer patients?' • 'What do *you* need to help you?' • Ground rules	Small group work & feedback
10.00	Learning priorities	Large group work & feedback
10.30	Break	
11.00	Theoretical perspectives (1) Psychosocial issues in cancer care	Didactic session
12.30	Reflecting on experience: 'How do people cope with cancer?'"	Small group work & feedback Brief didactic session on 'Coping with cancer'
13.00	Lunch	
13.30	Listening skills	Video demonstration
14.00	Assessment in cancer care	Role-play with simulated patient Course facilitators offer exemplar
15.00	Break	
15.15	'What have *we* learned so far?'	Large group work & feedback. Review of key issues
16.00	Agree structure for Day 2	
16.30	Close	
DAY 2		
09.00	Review Day 1 • Psychological care • Communication • Assessment	Group discussion
09.30	Review ground rules for role-play	Group discussion
09.45	Role-play 1: 'Dealing with difficult questions'	Role-play & feedback
10.30	Role-play 2: 'The angry patient'	Role-play & feedback
11.15	Break	
11.45	Role-play 3: 'Dealing with relatives' concerns	Role-play & feedback
12.30	Role-play 4: 'Dealing with collusion'	Role-play & feedback
12.15	Skills review: 'What have *we* learned so far?'	Group discussion
13.00	Lunch	
13.30	Role-play 5: 'Information giving'	Role-play & feedback
14.15	Role-play 6: 'Breaking bad news'	Role-play & feedback
15.00	Break	
15.30	The information needs of people with cancer	Didactic session
16.00	Skills review and evaluation	
16.30	Close	

Organisation of the learning experience

The use of actors, as simulated patients, provides a stimulating and refreshing approach to teaching communication skills with healthcare practitioners from a range of professional backgrounds, not least in the context of IPE. The particular strengths of this way of working reside in:

- the flexibility and versatility of the learning experience
- the opportunity to rehearse skills in a 'safe environment' that offers a convincingly real approximation of the clinical context (Donovan *et al*, 2003).

Although the focus in this chapter is on one short course designed to meet the needs of qualified, multiprofessional practitioners in the specific domain of cancer care, we have used this educational method in a variety of teaching contexts. These include pre-registration nursing programmes, post-qualification update courses, specialist practitioner preparation, and postgraduate clinical practice degree-level study. Although the content, learning outcomes, student experience and knowledge will vary in each case, common organisational issues can be identified in terms of maximising the value of the learning experience. Being well prepared is central to the success of this mode of learning, and thought needs to be given to how this is achieved in relation to both the student and the actor.

Student preparation

Regardless of the experience, discipline or status of students in terms of their own clinical practice, the prospect of participating in experiential learning involving simulated patients can be daunting and stress provoking (Burnard and Morrison, 1991). It is not untypically perceived simply as 'role-play' and accompanied by negative comments based upon exposure to what was often an unpleasant component of previous learning. Here, the facilitators need to be mindful of 'how' the subject is introduced to the learners, so that they engage in a productive way from the outset. When formulating timetable and module handbooks, or negotiating learning needs and resources with a student group, the language used is a key factor to consider. Although the use of simulated patients is becoming increasingly popular within medical and healthcare curricula, for many prospective students it is still 'new ground' with 'old anxieties'. Common responses to the introduction of 'experiential' involvement include:

> *'Do I have to take part'?*
> *'It's not real life.'*

> '*I do this sort of thing everyday, I'm good at it.*'
> '*I don't want to make a fool of myself in front of the others.*'
> '*I know my mind will just go blank.*'
> '*Can I just watch? I'll learn more that way.*'

Where the facilitator has the task of incorporating this method into an IPE initiative, the issues of group participation are compounded by the more insidious variables of professional-institutional power and authority. Those who see themselves as 'less important' in the professional hierarchy of healthcare (Freidson, 1970; Turner, 1987) may remain silent and, if not included immediately, 'split off' into a 'dissident' faction characterised by resentment or sabotage. Conversely, those with more 'senior' roles and responsibilities can feel embarrassed about exposing any perceived deficits in front of colleagues. These tensions are unlikely to be articulated as such, but require careful and sensitive handling if the obstacles are to be overcome. Based upon our experience, the following suggestions may be of assistance:

⌘ Formulation, at the outset, of shared 'ground rules' and group guidelines for ways of working together (see *Table 6.4*).

⌘ An opportunity for participants to explore their 'fears' combined with identification of individual 'strengths'.

⌘ Allowing time for the students to 'get to know each other', particularly in the context of some social activity or interaction.

Table 6.4: Examples of common 'ground rules'

❖ Respect each other's views

❖ Maintain confidentiality

❖ Allow individuals to have their say

❖ Participate fully in the programme

❖ Provide constructive feedback

❖ Allow 'time out' if issues become too emotionally laden

❖ Provide mutual support

If the above factors are taken into account, by the time the simulated patient is brought into the group the students should have established a sense of identity sufficiently cohesive to compensate for individual reservations. Peer support, reassurance, and collective problem-solving is vital to a successful experience, and need to be encouraged early in the programme as part of the group function. This can be enhanced by:

⌘ Introducing the model of communication teaching discussed previously as part of the orientation process, rather than 'pulling it out of the hat' later on (Parle *et al*, 1997).

⌘ Giving the students an opportunity to see how the model works in practice, with the facilitators taking 'patient' and 'practitioner' roles and the group participating to guide and steer the interaction.

⌘ Gradual involvement of group members by encouraging them to take part in exercises that are initially of short duration and require basic skills with which they are more likely to feel confident.

⌘ Allowing group members to 'experiment' with the types of roles to be used, before involving the simulated patient, so that they feel comfortable with the process.

⌘ Constructing scenarios that enable the students to interact with the simulated patient, as they would in their own professional role. In doing this, the students are not assigned a 'role to play' or a 'part to act' – they have only to be themselves.

Actor preparation

For the use of the simulated patient to be effective in both the learning experience and the achievement of learning outcomes, it is important that simulated patients are actively involved as part of the teaching team. This is as much in terms of planning as it is in the delivery of the session, where the actors will be visibly involved. The skill that the actor brings is one of 'breathing life' into a character that is one part of a clinical scenario designed to meet the learning needs of the students. The value of the simulated patient approach is that it captures the 'human spirit' of health care, and embraces the psychosocial dynamic of the 'human actor' in the broadest sense. It is therefore very different from other forms of teaching or assessment that rely, to one degree or another, on a quantitative system of measurement or marking. In making the optimum use of resources – practical, intellectual and creative – that the educator and actor can bring to any session, the following points have proved to be helpful:

⌘ Ensuring that the scenario and role are congruent with the 'lived experience' of the learners, and the intended outcomes of the session. This is more challenging, or complex, than it sounds, and is well worth the investment of time and effort. At this stage there is a need for close liaison between the actor, or his/her representative, and the course planning team – well in advance of the actual learning experience.

⌘ Facilitators need to be aware of what particular aspects of student skills they wish to focus upon – in this case, specific verbal and non-verbal components of interpersonal communication. To manage this effectively, the scenario needs to be constructed with attention to both the 'clinical' and 'emotional' make-up of patient–professional encounters. Examples are given in *Table 6.5*.

⌘ It is essential to arrange a 'briefing meeting' for actors and facilitators before the session, so that details can be discussed and 'flesh put on the bones' of the actor's character. Establishing appropriate characterisation is a crucial part of this process. It is insufficient for educators to focus on the 'clinical' picture, without helping the actor develop a unique persona to contextualise the scenario. Usually, the actor will also want to discuss the medical or clinical features of a particular 'condition' or 'treatment' that will inform the interaction. Likewise, the educator can explain the scenario's function, and the level of skill or expertise expected from the student.

⌘ Timing is also crucial to the success of the learning experience, as the use of simulated patients, though valuable, can be a costly item on educational budgets. Students need to be 'in the right place at the right time', and scheduled breaks must be rigidly adhered to. If all students are to benefit from the experience of participating, time slots need to be allocated and maintained. Where the simulated patient is being used in assessment strategies, such as the objective structured communication examination [OSCE] with large numbers of students, this issue assumes even greater prominence. Time should be apportioned at the close of the session for feedback, where the simulated patient ('in' or 'out' of role) is involved in an evaluation of the exercise.

⌘ Finally, consideration should be given to the 'scenery', 'props' and arrangement of furniture to 'set the scene' for each scenario (Burnard, 2002). Attention should be given to the size of the group, available and appropriate space, and the possible need for smaller 'syndicate' rooms.

Bespoke theatre in education

From the perspective of the actor, two conceptual definitions provide an important starting point for discussion of the role of the 'simulated patient' in interprofessional healthcare education (Sutton, 1998). Bespoke Theatre-in-Education [TIE] allows performing and devising skills to be put at the disposal of narrowly identified groups of clients who determine, and control, their own unique educational objectives and outcomes. Bespoke TIE has no 'ready-made' product (a show or play) and requires no audience as such. In 'content', and often in 'form', it is client specific. The actor/educator is the natural instrument for Bespoke TIE, and combines the performance skills of the actor with the communication, dialectical and evaluative skills of the educator. The actor/educator possesses the ability to:

- focus and contextualise issues by assimilating appropriate background information
- construct and respond to argument with convincing and controlled characterisations
- be flexible and proactive in performance
- contribute to learning outcomes
- provide detailed constructive feedback.

These definitions suggest two obvious and related applications. Bespoke TIE can be a valuable component of training, and the actor/educator is ideally qualified to contribute to courses and workshops dealing with various aspects of communication skills. The kind of work that the company, Actor/Educators Inc., provides for the Department of Nursing at the University of Liverpool and the local NHS trust involves a personal interaction between the actor as 'simulator' and the student or participant as 'role-player'. A simulator's function is to create a character in a situational model (scenario) designed for the practice or testing of necessary skills in the context of a training programme. As role-players, the students assume a role in preparation for future action or employment in the 'real world'. This important distinction means that actor/educators, normally, assume personalities and backgrounds very different from their own life experiences, whereas the student does not.

During the course of a simulation, actor/educators take responsibility for 'directing' the live scenario. They are able to manage the progression of the narrative and ensure that all of the specified learning, or assessment, issues are addressed. The actor can selectively exhibit behaviours in response to the stronger and weaker aspects of the students' practice. While it is axiomatic that actor/educators are convincing in their portrayal of character and situation to draw the role-player into their fiction, it is equally essential for there to be a part of their consciousness that functions as 'detached observer'. Without this, the actor/educator cannot manipulate a scenario, cannot give feedback and, in workshops, cannot respond to the interventions and directions of the facilitator.

It is important to understand that a simulated patient is both 'less', and 'more', than a real patient. 'Less' because the simulated patient is not suffering from the conditions or concerns portrayed, and the student knows this. 'More' because, by employing skills to promote a willing suspension of disbelief, the actor/educator consciously assists the learning or assessment process and, unlike the real patient, can be practised upon without sustaining 'damage'. In addition to the educational provision outlined above, actor/educators provide other distinct types of services. For example:

- ⌘ **Workshops:** In a healthcare context the actor presents as a simulated patient or relative, and in a veterinary context as a client. The patient/relative/ client is interviewed or consulted by one or more students while the rest of a small seminar group observes. The workshop is led by a facilitator who uses the actor as a versatile teaching resource, able to vary tone, attitude and direction in the interpretation of learning objectives as the interaction develops. Feedback 'in character', 'on behalf of the character', or both, is an essential component of workshop strategy. Extended workshops are designed to address broader or more long-term issues. Here, a single scenario, with intervals for feedback, discussion and forward planning, might last a whole teaching day. Workshops are utilised widely in undergraduate courses, but are also becoming a staple of heathcare in-service training.

⌘ **Objective structured communication examinations:** Actors take the part of a patient or relative, who will be interviewed by each candidate individually in the presence of an assessor. Here, the crucial requirement is consistency – to ensure that all candidates undergo the same assessment. Each student must therefore meet the same type of character with the same concerns and problems. Consistency between actors is attained through detailed briefing before the examination.

⌘ **Multimedia:** This includes training videos in the fields of cancer care, paediatric consultation and 'breaking bad news' training. Familiarity with healthcare issues is important in these projects.

⌘ **Demonstrations:** From time to time, actor/educators are invited to present communication skills scenarios to an audience of interested parties at conferences, or to illustrate a formal presentation. The method is the same as for a workshop, except that the interviewer is not in a learning situation and performance technique requires a greater emphasis on projection.

Assessment and evaluation

Although no formal assessment occurred within the programme described here, mounting evidence suggests that communication skills training, using a student-led agenda, enhances skill acquisition and translates into tangible improvements in practice (Wilkinson *et al,* 1999). The multiprofessional student-led approach, in this instance, certainly provided a valuable learning experience. An evaluation of the programme suggested that the students had gained new insights and perspectives from the opportunity to interact, and share their ideas, with other healthcare colleagues.

Table 6.5: Actors' and participants' briefing

STUDENT'S BRIEF

Fred Clifton is a 60-year-old man. He was diagnosed with cancer of the colon last year. He underwent an end-to-end anastomosis and made a good recovery. In the past few weeks he has become unwell again. A recurrence of the cancer is suspected. You are meeting Fred for the first time and you are required to undertake an assessment. For the purposes of the teaching programme, the assessment should not take longer than 15 minutes.

ACTOR'S BRIEF

You are Fred Clifton, a 60-year-old man. You are married to Sylvia. You have two children, Pauline and Michael, who are both married. They live locally and keep in touch. You retired from your job as a plumber when you became ill last year.

Personality and character
Before you were ill, you were a 'happy-go-lucky' sort of person. The cancer diagnosis 'knocked you for six' and you feel that you have never really recovered properly. The illness has made you a little more introspective and withdrawn. You used to enjoy playing snooker, but now you no longer go out as much as you did before your illness.

Medical history
Before your diagnosis you had been feeling 'off colour' and losing weight for several months. You went to the doctor when you noticed some blood in your stools. You were referred to the hospital, where you given the diagnosis. You had an operation to remove the cancer and recovered. You have been quite well until last month, when some of your original symptoms returned.

Psychological issues
You were 'very upset' at your diagnosis. Although you knew you were ill, you thought it might be some kind of inflammation. You did not expect to be told it was cancer. You recall your uncle dying from cancer 30 years ago and you have vivid memories of him 'fading away'. You strongly suspect that the cancer has returned and you are dreading receiving this news. You are feeling quite anxious and afraid. You have not had an opportunity to voice your fears to anybody yet. The extent of the worry has also lowered your mood lately. You are not sleeping or eating very well. You are also worried for your wife. You are particularly concerned about how she will cope if you become seriously ill or die.

Learning outcomes: The student should practise and develop:

- Prioritising key areas to cover during assessment

- Using appropriate question types

- Active listening skills

- Appropriate listening behaviours

- Strategies for dealing with 'difficult' questions

References

Burnard P, Morrison P (1991) Nurses' interpersonal skills: a study of nurses' perceptions. *Nurse Educ Today* **11**(1): 24–9

Burnard P (2002) *Learning Human Skills: An experiential and reflective guide for nurses and healthcare professionals.* 4th edn. Butterworth–Heinemann, Oxford

Department of Health (1995) *A Policy Framework for Commissioning Cancer Services. A report by the Expert Advisory Group on Cancer to the Chief Medical Officers of England and Wales (The Calman-Hine Report).* DoH, London

Department of Health (1999) *Making a Difference: Strengthening the nursing, midwifery and health visiting contribution to health and healthcare.* DoH, London

Department of Health (2000) *The NHS Cancer Plan.* DoH, London

Derogatis L, Morrow G, Fetting J, Penman D, Piatsky S, Schmale A (1983) Prevalence of psychiatric disorders among cancer patients. *JAMA* **249**: 751–7

Donovan T, Hutchison T, Kelly A (2003) Using simulated patients in a multiprofessional communications skills programme: reflections from the programme facilitators. *Eur J Cancer Care (Engl)* **12**: 123–8

Freidson E (1970) *Profession of Medicine: A study of the sociology of applied knowledge.* Dodd Mead, New York

Heaven C, Maguire P (1996) Training hospice nurses to elicit patient concerns. *J Adv Nurs* **23**: 280–6

Kruijver I, Kerkstra A, Bensing J, Van der Wiel (2000) Nurse/patient communication in cancer care: a review of the literature. *Cancer Nurs* **23**(1): 20–31

Maguire P, Faulkener A, Booth K, Elliot C, Hillier V (1996) Helping cancer patients disclose their concerns. *Eur J Cancer* **32A**: 78-81

Parle M, Maguire P, Heaven C (1997) The development of a training model to improve health professionals' skills, self-efficacy and outcome expectancies when communicating with cancer patients. *Soc Sci Med* **44**(2): 231–40

Reece I, Walker S (1997) *Teaching Training and Learning: A practical guide.* 3rd edn. Business Education Publishers, Sunderland

Sutton, R (1998) Supporting the bereaved relative: reflections on the actor's experience. *Med Educ* **32**: 622–29

Turner BS (1987) *Medical Power and Social Knowledge.* Sage, London

Wilkinson S (1991) Factors which influence how nurses communicate with cancer patients. *J Adv Nurs* **16**: 677-88

Wilkinson S, Bailey K, Aldridge J, Roberts A (1999) A longitudinal evaluation of a communication skills programme. *Palliat Med* **13**: 341–8

7

New NHS, new networks: a new agenda for promoting education for collaboration in cancer and palliative care

Anne Lanceley

Recent guidance from the NHS Executive (Department of Health [DoH], 1999) offers a long-term vision for continuing professional development that entails the cultivation of a learning environment in every health organisation to support lifelong learning within the framework of clinical governance. In addition, the circular recommends that opportunities for 'multidisciplinary and team-based learning' should increase, and scope for shared learning across health and social care should be explored. Departmental guidance also focuses on developing strategies for interprofessional work-based education. These challenges highlight the most pressing need for exponents of interprofessional education (IPE), which is to demonstrate how its content and learning methods can cultivate collaboration and teamwork in practice.

The chapter explores this challenge in the context of postgraduate cancer and palliative care education. A different sort of IPE will be discussed: one that may potentially lead to different outcomes — change in attitudes, heightened emotional capacity, reinforcement of collaborative confidence, and modification of individual and organisational behaviours — in ways that may be mutually reinforcing in benefiting patients. Where possible, exploration is supported by research evidence or description of work in progress. The discussion is underpinned by an examination of the values of educational practice in the fields of cancer and palliative care, and a link is made to contemporary practice and relationships between professionals.

The cancer and palliative care network agenda

There is a deep-seated shift in the NHS towards network-based forms of organisation and service delivery, and the future management of cancer services in the UK is set to occur within the context of managed care networks. During 1996 and 1997, practitioners working within cancer services became early adopters of the delivery network approach, based on a powerful medical case presented within *A Policy Framework for Commissioning Cancer Services* (Expert Advisory Group on Cancer, 1995). This report suggested that cancer centres, units and primary care teams should work in partnership with each other in network form, with patients being treated at the most appropriate level.

Care pathways between various providers need to be smooth for this model to work. The network model was a radical proposal at the time, given the then dominant model of the internal market, and was thought especially appropriate for cancer and palliative care because the care pathways of many people with cancer or other life-limiting illness are likely to be complex. The shift was essentially from a traditional vertical pattern of organising healthcare to a novel lateral model of organising.

The term 'managed network' implies that cancer and palliative networks may take a very different form from the tacit and self-regulated professional networks of the past. The question of whether such managed networks can promote the smoothly flowing care pathways envisaged has enormous practical implications for clinical practitioners, notably because key network building roles are undertaken not only by general managers but also by clinical-managerial hybrids such as clinical directors or 'lead clinicians' (Ferlie *et al*, 2002). These network builders may operate across local systems and face complex intra-organisational issues that demand organisational diagnostic skills — helpful in spotting likely areas of forward movement and change resistance.

Thirty-four cancer networks emerged after publication of *The NHS Cancer Plan* (DoH, 2000) and the majority of these are co-terminus with palliative care networks, the new strategic health authorities, and local county council boundaries. The cancer networks will coordinate commissioning from between seven and ten primary care trusts, making collaboration work at operational and strategic levels a significant management challenge.

The cancer and palliative networks were launched in advance of explicit consideration or research evidence of the styles of working required to support them, or the sort of education needed to develop staff (Lane *et al*, 2002; Taylor, 2002). As Loxley (1997) notes, collaboration has not been examined much either as a concept, in management terms, or as interprofessional clinical practice, although there is heavy usage of the term throughout the Calman–Hine report (1995).

Some empirical evidence for the characteristics and skills needed within network-based forms of NHS management are beginning to emerge. In their interview-based study, Ferlie and Pettigrew (1996) identified important concepts in use, as follows:

- trust
- reciprocity
- understanding
- credibility.

Achieving interorganisational trust might be considerably more difficult than building interpersonal trust, yet it is vital if alliances are to survive the departure of key individuals. The research highlights the important interpersonal psycho-emotional component to network-based forms of management. Implied in this and other more recent work (Pettigrew and Fenton, 2000) is that the shift to network-based forms of working may proceed over a long time frame, as the skills and learning capacity build up slowly. It is worth considering the nature of interprofessional collaboration in cancer and palliative care in more detail.

Interprofessional collaboration

'Interprofessional collaboration is a process not of incorporating the
knowledge and skills of others but of relating across boundaries, given
the differences between the professions. It is a device for managing
and organising resources and a technique for delivering services'
(Loxley, 1997: 90)

Interestingly, Ferlie and Pettigrew's (1996) concepts closely resemble the
conditions that Loxley identifies as vital for successful collaboration. For
example, Loxley talks about the trust required to work alongside others and
hand over responsibility to those with different training, competencies, and
competing priorities. Collaboration involves a willingness to contribute and to
receive contributions from others. This implies an acknowledgement that any
single perspective on the complex responses to cancer and palliative care need
is not all-encompassing. Collaboration, Loxley argues, is likely to be efficient
since it reduces the impact of unknown knowledge and unknown factors, and
increases reliability by enabling a wider understanding of meanings in cancer
and palliative care. For example, a previously active man with myeloma who
rejects adequate pain relief to help him maintain his activity has not, perhaps,
come to terms with his loss of a healthy body:

'I suppose in a way I'm worse off. I'm my own worst enemy in a way.
I ought to rest more than I do. I use the wheelchair and I stay in it
all day long, faithfully, and then I try and walk. I've got stiff and stuff
so I think, well, try being out of the chair a bit more and then you
get tired and you want to sit in the chair. And I don't know which end
of the candle to put out... I get depressed and I'm getting worse and I
don't know which way to go. What I'd like to do is just sort of ignore
the whole thing and get on with life, but I can't do that.'
(Lanceley, 1999)

The man's imaginative variation of burning the candle at both ends at once
represents and transfigures the essence of his predicament. Instead of 'burning
the candle at both ends', with its connotations of youthful energy, the man does
not know which end to put out in order to conserve his energy. He needs skilled
social work and counselling to help him maintain a balance between fighting
the illness and succumbing to its effects. Such input would also enable him to
make use of the range of skills of the cancer and palliative care team to help
alleviate his symptoms and distress.

Questions arise for interprofessional educationalists from Loxley's (1997) work and other ongoing empirical studies exploring the organisation and management of cancer services (Kewell *et al*, 2002). If the new lateral organisation is to become anything more than a veneer, laid on top of traditional vertical forms of organisation, professional groups need to be willing to share tasks with other professions in a broader way, rather than seek to defend their jurisdictions. As the cancer and palliative networks consolidate, there are important changes and implications for clinicians in terms of their professional development.

There has been a shift in the demands, expectations and attitudes of patients, and a growing recognition of the need for healthcare professionals to promote psychosocial wellbeing through working in partnership with patients. The UK has a reforming government with a commitment to patient-centred care as the keystone of its NHS reform programme. As the 'expert' patient/carer becomes a common phenomenon (Kendall, 2001), so professional roles will shift. A study by Barley *et al* (1999), designed to explore the needs of people with cancer for support and self-management, described many examples of unmet need. It recommended that healthcare professionals' education and training should address ways in which they can work collaboratively with people with cancer, and cushion them at the most vulnerable points in their cancer journey.

These shifts in perception and organisation need to be supported by education and training. As Ferlie *et al* (2002) argue, there is a need to develop a culture of reflective, undefended management and collaborative practice, conducive to egalitarian relationships. Yet, in practice the difficulties often experienced and described bear witness to irrationality, competition for power and resources, a defensive holding on to what is known, understood and practised, as well as defences against the distress inherent in cancer and palliative care. This chapter will examine these difficulties and consider the sort of IPE and training that might contribute to the development of collaborative forms of working in cancer and palliative care.

Professionals' experiences of working with people with life-threatening illness

A large body of work exists to suggest why it may be difficult for practitioners to remain open to the needs of dying patients (McNamara *et al*, 1995). Healthcare professionals struggle to process the difficult feelings they hear expressed every day, and while they may be adequately prepared in communication skills, they are ill equipped or lack confidence in their emotional capacity to deal with the powerful psychological trauma involved in working with people who have a life-threatening illness (Lanceley, 2001). This aspect of end-of-life care is considered important for any cancer and palliative care IPE initiative seeking to enhance the quality of care given to people with cancer and other life-threatening illnesses.

Exploration of the complexities of sustaining intensely demanding interpersonal relationships with people who have life-threatening illness is necessary if education and training are to have a sustained impact in practice. Such exploration of the 'underbelly' of practice has remained largely outside the influence of traditional education and training initiatives, and current literature suggests that it is likely to remain so (Taylor, 2002). Research in interprofessional communication skills training in cancer and palliative care over the past 20 years has shown that relatively short workshop-style training courses have the potential to enhance the skills of healthcare professionals (Heaven and Maguire, 1996). However, studies have not demonstrated that communication skills are maintained in practice at the same level over time (Parle *et al,* 1997). This raises obvious questions about the necessary balance at undergraduate and postgraduate level between teaching skills and attending to the attitudes, feelings and self-awareness of healthcare professionals needed to:

- effect and sustain communication with people with life-threatening illness
- develop trusting and sharing relationships with patients and professional colleagues.

It seems important to understand the context of communication and relationships with patients and colleagues; we need to understand how both healthcare professional and patient are grounded in and constrained by social conventions, institutional norms and procedure, and medical discourse (May, 1990).

The impact of cancer on healthcare professionals

There are conscious and unconscious processes at work in nurses' encounters with cancer, and fundamental issues about cancer nursing, to consider. These include:

- the distinctive aspects of interpersonal work
- how nurses use their personality on behalf of people for whom they are caring
- what the role imposes
- what irrational elements pertain
- the ways in which nurses communicate with patients and colleagues
- what nurses and patients may represent to each other
- how nurses manage their anxiety in the face of relentless pain and suffering.

(Lanceley, 2001: 100)

This view and the questions posed about the impact of cancer on nurses could equally be addressed to other members of the multidisciplinary team. What is important, as Corner (2002) notes, is that this view differs significantly from much writing, research and education in cancer and palliative care. It focuses on the ongoing nature of the work with patients rather than discrete encounters such as 'telling the diagnosis' or giving 'bad news', in which the healthcare professional (traditionally the doctor) tells and the patient responds. Instead nurses' day-to-day work is seen as 'interpersonal work'. In this context it acknowledges that relationships are socially and psychically constructed and exist within a wider organisational and social context. Furthermore, the nurse's conscious and unconscious feelings are acknowledged as an active part of the relationship, as is the burden of working in the intensely demanding environment of cancer care. The study highlights cancer nurses' reliance on self-protective stategies in their talk with patients. This is not a new finding, but an important and stable phenomenon in the field across a range of practitioners (McNamara, 1994; Froggatt, 1995; Lawton, 2000).

Acknowledging unconscious as well as conscious dimensions of cancer and palliative care is crucial if health and social care professionals are to develop their ability to work collaboratively with each other (Long, 2001) and in genuine partnership with patients and families affected by life-threatening illness.

The unconscious dimensions of care

An emphasis on the existence of unconscious processes and their role in interpersonal relations lies at the heart of psychodynamic understanding, which differs from other psychological theories primarily concerned with the conscious mind.

The unconscious dimensions of care involve early memories and feelings from the past that usually remain hidden from our conscious mind but can be triggered by something in the present. The impact of past memories on present behaviours can be a powerful one. A process of transference occurs, where thoughts and feelings, emotions and expectations belonging to a person in the past are transferred to a person in the present. That person is then reacted to as if he or she were the person from the past that is often inappropriate. An understanding of this process of transference may be an important tool in helping healthcare professionals to engage effectively with someone with a life-threatening illness and other relationships within the work setting.

Accurate identification of barriers to communication, and support and exploration of the complexities of sustaining intensely demanding interpersonal relationships with people with life-threatening illness, are necessary for training to have a sustained impact in practice. Such exploration has remained largely outside the influence of traditional training initiatives. Tinkering with interprofessional course content, while failing to look beneath the surface at the core of what healthcare workers do and how they do it, will not be sufficient to transform the professions and drive the patient-centred agenda. I will illustrate some tentative first steps in achieving this transformation from some 'work in progress'.

Work in progress

Experience of attending and then teaching on a short course entitled 'A psychodynamic understanding of cancer patients', developed by Ricky Emmanuel, Alexa Gilbert, David Sonnenberg and colleagues at the Tavistock Clinic, London, inspired my clinical and educational practice. Clear in my own mind of the relevance of the psychodynamic approach to cancer and palliative care, I sought to expand the scope of this original course through a robust educational partnership. I set out to achieve this partnership through a step-wise approach.

Step one: Recognition of need

The first step towards providing a different kind of postgraduate IPE was to form an alliance with another organisation that appeared to share some of the ideas described above. It is recognised that, if healthcare professionals are to acquire resilience and skills in sustaining attuned responses to people who have cancer and who are dying, postgraduate education for cancer and palliative care needs to be concerned with developing an understanding of emotional experience as well as teaching clinical skills for practice. An organisation local to me has this educational ethos and was a natural partner for the sort of educational initiative I had in mind.

Step two: Negotiation

Step two involved negotiation and discussion with highly experienced staff to consider the focus and delivery of a course that would broadly aim to provide a framework for understanding the emotional difficulties associated with cancer and palliative care work and the impact that this has on professional relationships. The most challenging aspect of these discussions was consideration of ways in which a spectrum of educational interventions could be used to ensure that learning would not be divorced from practice, but rather be based in the reality of the practice culture of cancer and palliative care. Collective experience and understanding of cancer and palliative care and the organisations in which it is practised and managed determined the educational approaches.

Step three: Defining content

Refining the formal academic component of the course was a relatively easy task in terms of content, since existing training provided by the partner organisation draws upon ideas of psychology, sociology, anthropology, psychoanalysis and family systems approaches. The course learning outcomes (*Table 7.1*) are being refined at the time of writing by an advisory group that includes a service user and a carer.

Table 7.1: Learning outcomes

⌘ Identification and use of personal reflection in order to learn from and enhance experience.

⌘ An awareness of the impact of unconscious communication in psychological support approaches.

⌘ An understanding of the team and institutional processes involved in close emotional contact and the impact on personal coping.

⌘ An understanding of the developmental issues regarding life-limiting illness throughout the individual life cycle.

⌘ An understanding of the unconscious processes that inform the cultural meanings and anxieties attached to disease and illness.

⌘ A critical appraisal of psychological assessment and ways of working with reactions to separation and loss.

⌘ A critical appraisal of psychological assessment and ways of working with reactions to separation and loss.

Step four: Learning activities

This step involved deciding on the amalgam of interventions to achieve the learning outcomes. With regard to the more formal classroom-based elements of the course, training would be in groups no larger than twenty so that an individual's voice and the group's capacity for reflection could be used as primary tools in the learning. The varied life and work experiences that individuals bring to the groups are valued as an important part of this learning. Students will be encouraged to develop their full potential through experiential learning in the classroom group and in work-based follow-up that reflects recent shifts in education.

Historically, nursing and medical education attempted to isolate and redefine interpersonal skills as technical skills and practices that can be imposed or acquired by education. This negates both the meaning that healthcare professionals attribute to communication and the emotional task of working with life-threatening illness, as well as their understanding of the conditions in which it takes place (May, 1990). To modify existing patterns of communication, healthcare professionals need to know what their current modes of communication accomplish, how feelings aroused by being with the patient may inform their communications more generally, and how they might think about this and adapt to certain situations and contexts.

Step five: Reflections on practice

Jarvis (1992) emphasises that reflection can lead to change in practice only when it includes the utilisation of theory and is supported by practice conditions. Equipping practitioners with a different way of thinking about their work in order to sustain the emotional task will not necessarily result in practice change. Students will need support and help in order to take this thinking into the workplace; consequently, flexible consultancy to involved trusts will be offered. This may take the form of 'learning from experience' seminars, learning sets and consultancy. Trust interest in these initiatives has been high.

Establishing interprofessional learning and teaching is often undermined by the boundaries set by professional and statutory body requirements of the curriculum and limited by the regulations of higher education institutions. This short course delivered on a part-time basis over one term is flexible, and at this stage in its development is not constrained by these regulations.

Conclusion

If healthcare professionals' anxieties can be sufficiently contained by the institution, through appropriate training, supervision or consultancy so that their distress is understood and they can articulate their painful experiences, they are more likely to engage in their work with cancer patients in a 'healthy' way (Menzies-Lyth, 1988; Obholzer and Roberts, 1994; Judd, 1995). Ironically, some forms of clinical supervision may function as a defence by ameliorating and smoothing over healthcare workers' ambivalent and difficult feelings concerning patients (Johns and Freshwater, 1998). However, if defence against anxiety, uncertainty and guilt is excessive, the patient's emotional needs cannot be 'heard' or met.

Healthcare professionals who work directly with patients and managers responsible for care pathways frequently cannot make the patient better. Some denial and defensiveness is inevitable on the part of the healthcare worker and the patient, but a healthy cancer and palliative care context is one where enough individuals continue to struggle to admit their more primitive fantasies, emotions and helplessness and, by owning them, can better contain the patient's helplessness. The sort of IPE described in this chapter would go some way to helping healthcare professionals to do this, with and for each other for the benefit of patients. One thing is clear: to simply try harder within existing frameworks and paradigms is, to echo Sheldon and Smith (1996), 'a mistaken use of energy'.

References

Barley V, Tritter J, Daniel R (1999) *Meeting the Needs of People with Cancer for Support and Self-management*. A collaborative project between Bristol Oncology Centre, Department of Sociology, University of Warwick, and Bristol Cancer Help Centre Report. Presented at Highgrove House, Tetbury

Corner J (2002) Nurses' experiences of cancer. *Eur J Cancer Care* **11**: 193–9

Department of Health (1999) *Continuing Professional Development: quality in the new NHS*. Health Service Circular 1999/154. NHS Executive, Leeds

Department of Health (2000) *The NHS Cancer Plan: A plan for investment. A plan for reform*. DoH, London

Expert Advisory Group on Cancer (1995) *A Policy Framework for Commissioning Cancer Services* (The Calman–Hine Report). Department of Health, Wales

Ferlie E, Pettigrew A (1996) Managing through networks: some issues and implications for the NHS. *British Journal of Management* **7** (Special Issue): 81–99

Ferlie E, Hawkins C, Kewell B (2002) Managed networks within cancer services: an organizational perspective. In: James R, Miles A (Eds). *Managed Care Networks: Principles and practice*. Aesculapius Medical Press, London: 1–13

Froggatt K (1995) Nurses and involvement in palliative care work. In: Richardson A, Wilson-Barnett J (Eds). *Nursing Research in Cancer Care*. Scutari Press, London: 151–64

Heaven CM, Maguire P (1996) Training hospice nurses to elicit patient concerns. *J Adv Nurs* **23**: 280–6

Jarvis P (1992) Reflective practice and nursing. *Nurse Educ Today* **12**: 174-81

Johns C, Freshwater D (Eds) (1998) *Transforming Nursing through Reflective Practice*. Blackwell, Oxford

Judd D (1995) *Give Sorrow Words: working with a dying child*. Whurr, London

Kendall E (2001) *The Future Patient*. Institute for Public Policy Research, London

Kewell B, Hawkins C, Ferlie E (2002) Calman-Hine reassessed: a survey of cancer network development in England, 1999–2000. *J Eval Clin Pract* **8**(3): 303–11

Lanceley A (1999) The patient and nurse in emotion talk and cancer: 'the tempest in my mind.' Unpublished PhD thesis, University of London

Lanceley A (2001) The impact of cancer on healthcare professionals. In: Corner J, Bailey C (Eds). *Cancer Nursing: Care in context*. Blackwell Science, Oxford: 100–19

Lane C, Kelly C, Clarke D (2002) Cancer networks: translating policy into practice. In: Clarke D, Flanagan J, Kendrick K (Eds). *Advancing Nursing Practice in Cancer and Palliative Care*. Palgrave, Basingstoke

Lawton J (2000) *The Dying Process: Patient experiences of palliative care*. Routledge, London

Long S (2001) Working with organizations: the contribution of the psychoanalytic discourse. *Organisational and Social Dynamics* 2: 174–95

Loxley A (1997) *Collaboration in Health and Welfare: Working with difference*. Jessica Kingsley, London

McNamara B, Waddell C, Colvin M (1995) Threats to the good death: the cultural context of stress and coping among hospice nurses. *Sociol Health Illn* 17(2): 222–44

May C (1990) Research on nurse-patient relationships: problems of theory, problems of practice. *J Adv Nurs* 15: 307–15

Menzies-Lyth I (1988) The functioning of social systems as a defence against anxiety. In: *Containing Anxiety in Institutions: selected essays*. Free Association Books, London: 43–94

Obholzer A, Roberts VZ (Eds) (1994) *The Unconscious at Work: Individual and organizational stress in the human services*. Routledge, London

Parle M, Maguire P, Heaven C (1997) The development of a training model to improve health professionals' skills, self-efficacy and outcome expectancies when communicating with cancer patients. *Soc Sci Med* 44(2): 231–40

Pettigrew A, Fenton E (2000) *The Innovating Organization*. Sage, London

Sheldon F, Smith P (1996) The life so short, the craft so hard to learn: a model for post-basic education in palliative care. *Palliat Med* 10: 99–104

Taylor R (2002) Postgraduate medical education for modern cancer services. In: Baker MR (Ed). *Modernising Cancer Services*. Radcliffe Medical Press, Abingdon: 131–51

8

Organic training and development: working with mental health teams directly in the workplace

Mick McKeown, Phil Blundell, Julie Lord and Caroline Haigh

In this chapter we develop the argument that progressive changes to routine practice are best effected through a process of working with whole teams together, directly, in the workplace. We draw upon interprofessional initiatives that we have been involved in to illustrate an underpinning philosophy, which we refer to as 'organic training and development'. The lessons learnt from our attempts to evaluate such projects are offered to highlight a number of issues that are more likely to indicate successful team-learning and associated practice development.

Our main focus has been on teams of staff working in various inpatient mental health settings — a clinical domain that has been the subject of pointed recent criticism, and hence constitutes an interesting point of departure for efforts towards concerted practice change. Not least of the criticisms has been a bemoaning of the inability of traditional approaches to training to address real change in routine clinical practice. The chapter proceeds with a discussion of our most recent project, targeted at enhancing the degree of service user involvement in routine care on an acute mental health ward. Here we describe the use of techniques of non-participant observation of routine working to evaluate effectiveness. We conclude with some observations on the difficulties in properly funding this sort of project.

The critique of inpatient mental health practice

Mental health services in general, and inpatient provision in particular, have been the subject of almost continuous critique and policy prescription for the past decade or more (Department of Health [DoH] 1994; Clinical Standards Advisory Group Committee on Schizophrenia, 1995; Mental Health Act Commission and the Sainsbury Centre, 1997; DoH, 1999; Standing Nursing and Midwifery Advisory Committee [SNAMC], 1999). In recent years a growing body of formal and informal evidence has suggested that mental health inpatient services are being stretched to the limits, are unable to meet minimum standards of care, are understaffed, and are providing services that are both unsafe and non-therapeutic. Specific criticisms include the poverty of therapeutic environment in mental health wards, and the lack of systematic involvement of people with mental health problems in their own care. The

SNAMC report into acute inpatient mental health settings (1999: 9–10) stated:

> '... *inpatient units are becoming increasingly custodial in their atmosphere. Our work suggests that users in acute care often feel that they are being deprived of therapeutic activity, have much less contact with nurses than they would wish, and at times feel unsafe... Despite the fact that there are now a wide range of evidence-based... interventions which could be a component of inpatient care, these are rarely used by nurses. Apart from a few exemplary programmes, no training in evidence-based interventions is available to the majority of nurses working in inpatient settings.'*

Interestingly, the SNMAC report (1999) also highlighted practitioner dissatisfaction with a perceived distant relationship between universities and health trusts, which was felt to compromise education and training initiatives. The authors of the report linked such concerns with a call for more work-based training for all staff.

In addition to the official voice of criticism found in these reports, service-users themselves are rightly demanding improved quality of care when they need to be admitted to hospital. The progressive growth of the user movement has highlighted the relative lack of involvement of individuals in their own care, leading to calls for more participatory services (Rogers *et al*, 1993; Perkins and Repper, 1996) based upon therapeutic alliances (Frank and Gunderson, 1990) influencing recent policy (DoH, 2001a,b). The current government's strategy, acknowledging service failings, sets out to ensure that services are wide-ranging, accessible, of therapeutic value and available when needed. This not only provides an opportunity to address longstanding problems in acute inpatient care, but also presents the challenge of bringing about substantial change in a complex and hard-pressed sector of care.

The gap between the aspirations of the National Service Framework and the day-to-day reality of much acute inpatient care, however, remains significant. It was against this background that, in 1998, the Centre for Mental Health Services Development, Kings College London, launched the Acute Inpatient Practice Development Network, a two-year project that aimed to improve the quality of the inpatient experience for service users.

Traditional education for mental health staff

Arguably, the highlighted problems facing acute mental health settings are antithetical to the policy goal of enhancing evidence-based practice. The sort of clinical interventions that do have an established evidence base have either been researched in simpler contexts than inpatient wards, or would require, for their systematic implementation, the sort of therapeutic environment that is felt to be lacking in these environments. Crucially, a number of commentators have pointed out that practitioner skills deficits contribute to the failure to offer a range of effective therapies, yet traditional models of training have negligible impact at the level of services, whatever the quality of individual programmes (Fadden, 1997; McKeown *et al*, 2000). Gournay and Sandford (1998) argue that much of the available research regarding the effectiveness of education and training is of limited value, and that large-scale controlled evaluations are necessary.

A major problem with traditional models of practitioner training is that all too often one or two members of a team receive training, usually in a university classroom away from the workplace, and are then expected to return and establish new knowledge and skills into their routine care provision. More often than not, services are not best organised to facilitate such a contribution to practice change, and an unfair burden is placed on these individuals. Typically, various organisational impediments conspire to ensure that plans for implementing new ways of working are stillborn, expose existing tensions in team-working, and result, if anything, in a deterioration in staff morale.

An interesting illustration of such a scenario is provided by the national efforts to train practitioners in psychosocial interventions for people with serious mental health problems. The available training is of demonstrably high quality, typified in the Thorn and COPE (Collaboration on Psychosocial Education) initiatives (Gournay and Sandford, 1998; Lancashire *et al*, 1996; Rolls *et al*, 2002), yet the uptake of specific therapeutic interventions into routine practice, despite the training of large numbers of practitioners, has been extremely limited. This led Fadden (1998: 177) to assert:

> *'The fact that effective treatments are available but are not being offered is unjustifiable on moral or ethical grounds. If the present situation is to change, the main focus must be on developing successful methods of disseminating these interventions into ordinary clinical services. The issues to be addressed are training of clinicians, ongoing supervision and monitoring of skills acquired, and how service systems need to change to facilitate this type of work.'*

Collaborative working and interprofessional learning on mental health wards

If we consider mental health services as a whole, then failures of team-working, particularly in terms of effective communication, figure highly in the most pointed critiques. Such negative factors, together with the general need to improve the quality of care for service users and make more efficient use of resources, lend support to the emergent 'bandwagon' to promote collaborative multiprofessional working (Mackay *et al*, 1995).

Collaborative working within mental health services has been a government aim since the 1970s (Couchman, 1995) and has been emphasised in a number of government reports spanning the past two decades (Department of Health and Social Services [DHSS,] 1980; DoH 1990, 1994, 1995, 1996, 1997, 1998). Interprofessional learning is generally seen as a key way to promote more effective team-working and collaboration (WHO, 1988; NHSE, 1996) and is increasingly prominent within published policy and guidance of relevance to mental health teams (Sainsbury Centre for Mental Health, 1997; DoH, 2000) and acute wards in particular (SNMAC, 1999; DoH, 2002). Although national recommendations challenge the various professions to move beyond traditional educational models, very few programmes have acknowledged the value of pursuing future-orientated multiprofessional approaches with whole teams within their own workplace.

Henneman *et al* (1995) define collaboration as:

> '...a process by which members of various disciplines share their expertise.'

However, a great deal of confusion surrounds the terminology of relevant learning, with 'interprofessional', 'multiprofessional', 'shared' and 'collaborative' all being used interchangeably along with other terms. Hammick (1998) distinguishes between the terms 'multiprofessional' and 'interprofessional', describing the former as 'learning together' and the latter as 'learning together to promote collaborative practice'.

Despite the importance attached to the achievement of collaboration, it would appear that this is the exception rather than the rule in most practice settings (Henneman *et al*, 1995). The degree to which collaboration and effective team-working are practised within mental health services, in particular, is affected by a number of limiting factors (Reeves, 2001). Various studies, focused mainly on the practices of community mental health teams, highlight the challenges to collaborative working (Beattie, 1995; Couchman, 1995; Griffiths 1997; Norman and Peck, 1999). Such challenges include:

- different professional cultures and associated loyalties
- allegiance to dissimilar conceptual frameworks for understanding the needs of service-users

- attachment to differing approaches to care and treatment
- conflict arising from aspects of the division of labour, notably clinical leadership and lines of accountability and responsibility.

Mackay *et al* (1995) posited the qualities necessary for individuals to effectively practise interprofessional collaboration, indicating the enormity of realising this in healthcare settings. These practitioners would have to be brave enough to locate themselves outwith the safety and protection of their own professional group and be willing to listen to the views of others, valuing and acknowledging the contribution they make. Attempts to achieve this would:

> '...reflect a maturity of perspective lacking in most areas of
> enterprise in the late twentieth century.'
>
> (Mackay *et al*, 1995: 10)

Many advocates of interprofessional learning see it as a means of promoting collaborative working across a variety of health and social care settings (for example, Mathias and Thompson, 1997; Headrick *et al*, 1998), suggesting that it offers the opportunity to:

- avoid professional stereotyping and negative attitudes towards other disciplines (Carpenter and Hewstone 1996, DePoy *et al*, 1997)
- improve communication and teamwork between the various professions (Van der Horst *et al*, 1995; Virgin *et al*, 1996)
- ensure a clearer understanding of roles and achieve common goals (Richardson and Edwards, 1997; Reeves, 2000).

Cook (1995) argues that these positive effects accrue from shared contact in the learning process.

Cautionary voices criticise a lack of conceptual clarity, robust supporting evidence, and uncertainty about how to proceed (for example, Campbell, 1999; Barr, 2000; Glenn, 2002). Finch (2000) suggests that higher education institutions need a clearer policy lead than is currently available to be able to plan for comprehensive and systematic programmes of interprofessional learning, asking the question: what exactly does the NHS really want? Glenn (2002) progresses similar themes to urge a realistic view of what can be achieved by interprofessional education (IPE) strategies, remarking that these cannot substitute for other forms of consultation in workplaces where tensions are evident. She points out that the task of IPE is complicated by the fact that current professional roles and boundaries are under review in a climate of flexible working.

Finch (2000) observes that much of the commentary about IPE appears to assume that this learning will take place in university classrooms. She goes on to argue that it would be a more effective use of resources, though an organisational challenge, to envisage interprofessional learning taking place directly in the clinical setting. Arguably, when shared learning or IPE is applied within the clinical settings, a degree of collaboration and a commitment to teamwork are essential prerequisites.

Stark and colleagues (2002) conclude from their large study of teamwork in mental health that there remains a gap between the rhetoric of terms such as multiprofessional, interprofessional, and interdisciplinary working and the reality of complex, contradictory and vexed team-working in practice. They caution against the feasibility of providing idealised blueprints for team-working that do not acknowledge cultural and political contingencies at grass-roots level. This leads to a persuasive assertion that attention to team-working in education must relate to the real context, and avoid definitive prescriptions for behaviour. In this respect, Stark *et al* (2002: 417) point out that the problem with team-working is not necessarily a lack of knowledge of appropriate theory, but rather the emotional labour that goes with attempting to work effectively as a team in trying circumstances:

> *'Mental healthcare seems to suffer less from under-informed minds than from mismanaged hearts. And "hearts", [we] would argue, are even less susceptible to universal prescription than minds.'*

Miller and colleagues (2001) propose a model for multiprofessional education grounded in a shared learning approach that utilises client-based scenarios to foster knowledge acquisition and team-working. They envisage a range of applications for this approach, including 'whole-team learning', where it is important to address scenarios that are based on the actual team-working context. By jointly working through relevant scenarios the team can meet a number of learning objectives, including developing:

- an agreed philosophy and culture
- structures of team-working strategies for clinical intervention
- systems for induction of new team members
- patterns of communication within the team.

(Miller *et al*, 2001)

A recently conducted systematic review of studies into the effects of IPE involving practitioners caring for adults with mental health problems was carried out as part of the preliminary activity for a 'National Demonstration Project' (see below). This review concluded that the evidence was patchy (Reeves, 2001). Only 19 studies were found with the relevant focus (only three UK studies), raising questions concerning the translation of findings to unlike cultural and organisational settings. Other deficiencies in the reviewed papers included methodological shortfalls, insufficient detail in the descriptions of the education programmes, and a lack of emphasis upon service-user outcomes. Seven of the papers utilised a methodologically weak, quantitative post-intervention design, with no collection of baseline data. Some of the better-designed studies either reported upon projects that involved relatively short educational interventions or restricted outcome measures to those of limited value, such as client satisfaction. Furthermore, only four of the studies employed a longitudinal research design, leaving open the question of the extent to which the effects of interprofessional learning persist beyond the completion of the intervention (Reeves, 2001).

The process of organic training and development

It is our contention that an organic approach to interprofessional training and development is one way of addressing these concerns, because the goal of changing systems is integral to the process. It is not just the content of training and education that needs attention: the process is of equivalent importance if the aim is to effect significant change in the practice and organisation of teams. If this is indeed the case, then concomitant evaluations should also address process variables.

The approach that we advocate takes place directly in the clinical environment within which any changes to practice have to occur, and targets the learning needs of whole teams working together. The goal is that team training and practice development are enacted simultaneously in an 'organic' process of transformation. Mutual respect for the different forms of expertise brought to the interaction between trainers and clinical staff is fostered, and their skills and knowledge are synthesised in developing new forms of practice that are much more likely to endure beyond cessation of the training input.

The organic approach has been developed in response to the challenges to implementing progressive change in inpatient environments, and shares some common ground with other initiatives that have been designed to address similar problems. Essentially, these approaches attempt to incorporate lessons from the field of organisational psychology to the endeavour of effecting enduring developments in routine practice.

Corrigan and McCracken's (1995, 1997) process of interactive staff training (IST) emphasises both working with entire teams and training in the actual workplace where practice change has to be delivered. In their exposition of the IST approach, Corrigan and McCracken (1995) articulate a vision of trainers with particular expertise that is new to the team, meeting with staff who are acknowledged as experts in their own working environment. Working together they adapt the new knowledge to best suit the contingencies of everyday practice. This respectful stance towards the host team is resonant with the appreciative inquiry approach to organisational change (Cooperrider and Srivastva, 1987), wherein any problems are understood constructively, and practice development commences with an appreciation of individual and collective strengths, rather than damagingly focusing on weaknesses.

With a view to tackling systems, Corrigan and McCracken (1995) list three main obstacles to establishing improvements in inpatient settings that have been described in relevant research:

⌘ Bureaucratic constraints, including practitioner time taken up in administrative tasks and inability or unwillingness to properly fund appropriate programmes of care.

⌘ Scientific reporting of innovative treatment interventions that lack clarity or meaning to grass-roots staff, raising questions over the accessibility of effective treatments to practitioner teams.

⌘ Insufficient numbers of well-trained personnel to deliver innovative programmes.

The IST approach was developed in the US for training teams to practise behavioural interventions for psychiatric rehabilitation, and has been evaluated with encouraging results (Corrigan *et al,* 1997). Appreciative inquiry was also developed as an approach in the US and has been undertaken in a number of diverse settings, including modern businesses and community development projects. Latterly, the approach has been instigated in the UK, with a notable initiative in the Prison Service (Liebling *et al,* 1999). Appreciative inquiry is grounded in principles of action research and is well suited to this form of evaluation. If whole-team training is to become an accepted format for practice development, then effective methods of evaluation are required. Previous work in this respect raises the potential for eclectic use of both experimental research designs and action research methods, perhaps mixing these within single projects.

Milne *et al* (2002) report on a promising pilot study that focused on the issue of transfer of learning into practice. Education that included an element of relapse prevention training, aimed at 'immunising' participants against prevailing barriers to the generalisation of learning into practice, was compared with a short standard programme of training in psychosocial interventions for multidisciplinary mental health staff. The relapse prevention component included attention to raising awareness of the obstacles to implementation of learning, and concepts and strategies of goal setting, group problem-solving and coping skills. Although outcome measures were limited to self-report questionnaires for the participating staff, these produced interesting findings. The group who received the relapse prevention training reported significantly greater generalisation of learning into practice, yet there were no significant differences between the two groups in terms of reaction to the training or perceptions of the barriers they faced.

The North West Region NHS Executive recently funded a National Demonstration Project for competency-based training in adult mental health care, delivered by the University of Central Lancashire (with PB and MM involved as trainers) and independently evaluated by the University of Bradford. This two year, part-time modular course used interactive methods to train whole teams of staff. A number of community mental health teams and inpatient teams from across the northwest of England were involved, and were allocated to one of two distinct training formats. These comprised a 'time-out' model, wherein the team would come together for classroom-based learning for one afternoon every fortnight, and a 'debriefing' model, which involved the training facilitators working a complete shift with the team. The debriefing process would conclude with a meeting of participants to reflect on the day's events in relation to the course learning objectives.

Both interventions were concerned with individual student attainment, and also collective engagement in thinking through team applications of learning. In one sense, the debriefing model has similarities with scenario-based learning (Miller *et al,* 2001) in that case-examples inform the learning process, with these having the benefit of indisputable authenticity and immediacy of structured engagement in learning.

The evaluative review of this project has yet to be published, but it is worth noting here the importance of effective managerial support to the success or failure of programmes of this kind. Those sites where managerial attention to site selection, preliminary work to ensure a perception of team ownership and choice in involvement in the project, and workforce issues, such as strategies for maximising attendance and supporting additional study time, were likely to see the most successful outcomes.

All of these approaches have in common the fact that process issues are emphasised, drawing on various theories of organisational change. Obviously the content of any training input is important, but how learning is associated with changing practice is paramount. There is a synthesis of any new knowledge brought by the trainers/facilitators with the grass-roots expertise held by the individual participants. Essentially, new practices emerge from a collaborative effort to shape and adapt what is learnt to better fit the actual environment. The ultimate aim is for any positive developments to be self-sustaining. Any changes to working practices are then more likely to last after the trainers leave, and become incorporated into daily routines.

The focus is on collective groups, rather than seeing learning as the province of individual students. There is a similar concern with collective outcomes and ownership of these. The whole teams of staff or community groups are targeted, with collaborative working proceeding directly in the environment wherein specific developments are sought. The philosophical starting point is to understand, rather than condemn, any visible faults or difficulties within the host group, and, most importantly, to highlight the positive aspects. Given the often beleaguered situation that typifies inpatient mental health units, this strategy is timely. Interestingly, from a psychosocial perspective there is an analogue here with behavioural family therapy, wherein the therapists seek to understand the challenges faced by families and foster an affirming style of feedback and interaction, and eventual autonomy in effective problem-solving.

Particularly if we think of modern health services, the principles of organisational psychology tell us that ownership of ideas and practice developments is vital. However, it is often the case that readymade blueprints for practice change are imposed on staff, with predictable and disappointing outcomes. The alternative allows for a style of service development that grows 'organically' towards individual, collective and organisational improvements to services that may not have been anticipated in advance. This process has been described as organic because the practice developments have their origins in the team themselves, and must turn out to be suited to the practice environment because they have been shaped to that end.

Organic training in practice

We have been involved in a number of organic training initiatives, two of which we will describe briefly here to illustrate some simple lessons that can be drawn from the experiences that may usefully inform future, similar IPE projects.

A project at Rathbone Hospital in Liverpool aimed to train the team in psychosocial approaches to the care of individuals with severe and enduring mental health problems, in the context of a secure rehabilitation ward. The project is reported upon at greater length elsewhere (McKeown *et al,* 2000, 2002) and was interesting for a number of reasons. First, there was an established and extensive multidisciplinary team focused exclusively on this unit, which is not necessarily typical of other inpatient care. Importantly, key members of the team were committed and enthusiastic towards the aims of the project and were thoroughly involved at all stages. The training facilitators were 'of the team', comprising a clinical psychologist and a nurse lecturer-practitioner (MM), both trained in the theory and practice of psychosocial interventions. Camsooksai (2002) has highlighted the benefits of the lecturer-practitioner role in the context of IPE.

The organic process at Rathbone resulted in a number of positive outcomes, all of which involved changes to the practice and organisation of team-working. The challenge of adopting and adapting psychosocial approaches into routine practice caused the team to scrutinise the way they organised such work as record keeping and case-reviews. It became clear that the current routines and practices were not best suited to effective team-working. Individual members of the multidisciplinary team did not fully understand, or even typically see, each other's notes and records, and the overall quality of certain records mitigated against effective retrieval of relevant information. These factors led the team to work together to construct new systems, including a shift to a psychosocial model of care to inform the whole team's practice (Savage and McKeown, 1997), and a process of whole-team care planning with a single, multidisciplinary case record (McKeown *et al,* 2000, 2002).

Our most recent project was undertaken at an acute mental health ward in Leigh Infirmary which was signed up to the national Acute Inpatient Practice Development Network. The project team comprised two nurse lecturers (PB and MM), the local practice development nurse (JL) and a research assistant (CH). The focus of the training was to foster the development of ward-based initiatives to enhance the degree of involvement and participation of service users in their own care, and this took place over a six-month period. The training involved an initial 'away-day' session, followed by one day a week ward-based activity akin to the debriefing model described earlier.

The evaluation was designed as a pilot study and comprised baseline measures of staff and client variables (pre-training), interim staff measures (immediately post-training), and staff and client measures at six-month follow-up. The staff outcomes were measured by questionnaires, focusing on relevant knowledge, self-assessment of relevant competencies and attitudes towards service-user involvement. Service-user outcomes were measured by questionnaires that focused on self-efficacy, social behaviour, satisfaction, and perceptions of the ward environment. Forty service users were recruited at baseline, and twenty at follow-up (the latter recruitment was hampered by closure of the ward for refurbishment). A purposive sample of staff and service users at baseline and at follow-up participated in qualitative interviews to explore perceptions of ward life in relation to user involvement; staff were also asked about reaction to the training process.

Reeves (2001) argues that many IPE evaluations are of limited value because little attention is afforded to process measures that would offer insight into how change occurs. Observational measures are suggested as one possible way of tackling this shortfall. In our study we employed a process of non-participant observation of key aspects of ward routine, which were undertaken at baseline, interim and follow-up. We were interested in the extent and quality of service user participation, or staff use of language indicative of their acknowledgement of user perspectives. We chose to look at ward rounds and nursing shift handovers (as occassions where team members gathered collectively) and medication dispensation times (as situations resonant with opportunities to engage with clients over an important clinical issue). Initially, we observed these interactions informally to get a feel for the sort of speech typically transacted. From field notes we constructed categories of interaction that could be measured by simple frequency counts. For the ward rounds we also conducted a time budget of which individuals were speaking over a period of one hour from the commencement of the meeting. Four ward rounds, four medication rounds and four handovers were observed at each interval, with the data aggregated in the results.

The results of these observations for the medication dispensing times are shown in *Figure 8.1*. As can be seen, over the period of the project there was a shift in the sort of communication undertaken in this context, evidenced most prominently at the interim stage, but persisting at follow-up. At baseline, the nurse dispensing medication mainly engages in talk that does not have medication as its focus, there is relatively little direct eliciting of service-user concerns or of service users raising their own concerns. As the project proceeded, there is more emphasis in these interactions on medication and side-effects, and the service users themselves become less passive, and spontaneously bring up their own issues. All of these outcomes were in line with the aims of the training programme.

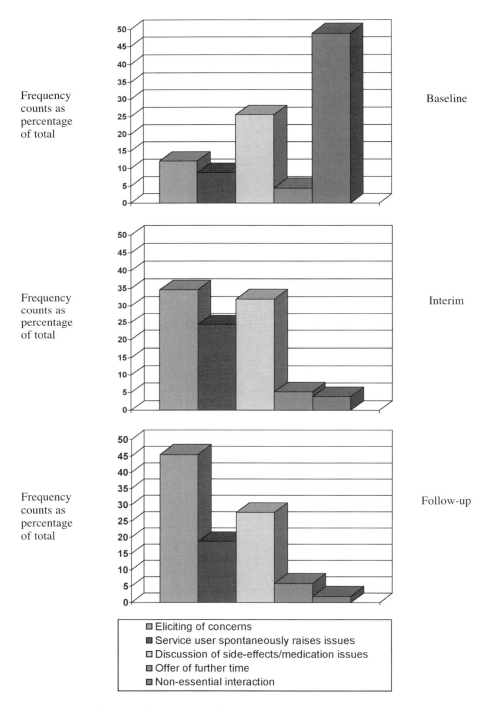

Figure 8.1: Medication dispensing observations at baseline, interim and follow-up

The results of the observations of the nursing shift handovers showed similar changes, with a shift towards talk that indicated a focus on service-user perspectives, more active participation of all nurses in the discussions, and inclusion of more supportive and constructive contributions. The ward round observations were less clear-cut, and the aggregation of the data served to hide marked differences between the rounds involving different consultant psychiatrists. On a positive note, there was a general shift towards more encouragement of service-user opinion, although there was little evidence that service users themselves became more actively involved in these meetings, and professional staff discourse dominated the time-budgets.

In one sense, the relative lack of service-user involvement promoted in ward rounds could reflect a general dissatisfaction with the format and organisation of this type of case-focused meeting. Service users may prefer to meet their team and voice concerns in different settings or circumstances. However, the relative lack of impact in an extant and important part of ward routine may be better explained in terms of the extensiveness of involvement of the whole team in the project, and associated power differences. In the course of the project it was clear that, for whatever reasons, it was only the nursing staff who were fully engaged. Although various disciplines, notably social workers and community nurses, attended the initial away day, only the ward-based nurses got involved in the ward-based element of the training. The ward psychiatrists did not take direct part in any of this activity. Hence, any attempt to organically grow new working practices was dependent on those staff who were active participants attempting to influence others who were not actively engaged in the whole. This was a less than satisfactory state of affairs, bearing unfavourable comparison with Rathbone where a range of disciplines was actively involved, including the unit psychiatrist.

Although this project incorporated some elements of an action research approach, perhaps a more thorough appraisal of the practice setting, particularly an examination of the team dynamics before commencing the learning component, would have been useful. Patient care rounds offer an excellent opportunity to assess the presence or absence of collaboration within a team (King *et al*, 1993). An essential requirement for this approach to learning is that the team is fundamentally non-hierarchical and willing to share power, knowledge and expertise. The dominance of certain professional groups and the failure of key individuals to make substantial contributions within the meeting may be indicative of a hierarchical team that may not always value a joint approach to working, sharing of leadership, or a respect for fellow team members. The observation element of this project may have been the first structured examination of the processes and dynamics within this particular team.

The restriction of participation in the training element to nurses does help to illustrate the versatility of nurses in the context of organisational change. Although the mental health nurse is often perceived as a skilled generalist and a 'jack of all trades', it can be argued that a positive side to this is a willingness to take on new initiatives and to attempt to break down professional boundaries. In effect, we were reliant upon the ward nurses to take up the challenge presented by the project and be catalysts for change across the whole team. There is evidence from the observations that this was achieved to some degree.

The future

The lack of a truly multidisciplinary involvement in the Leigh project is open to explanation in terms of the very commentary that provides the rationale for interprofessional learning in the first place, and at least in part could say something about the initial extent of progressive team-working in place. Evans and Carlson (1992) assert that collaboration requires an environment with an existing team orientation. Such observations lead us to conclude that the ability of any team to engage with a process of interprofessional learning should not be taken for granted, and that such programmes may need to incorporate initial or ongoing activity designed to promote particular knowledge and skills compatible with a collaborative approach. It would be advisable, at the commencement of such projects, for all team members to establish ground rules to address issues such as non-attendance at teaching sessions, along with individual and collective responsibilities. It may also be germane to allocate more preparatory time to socialise the staff into the principles and ethos of the organic learning process and the action elements of the research evaluation. This would be analogous to Harrison and Kitchens' (1989) notion of research facilitation, whereby staff are motivated and initiated into involvement in research projects.

It is also important to recognise that attendance is also dependent upon any operational constraints that may affect the programme. In practice, many of the problems associated with bringing the various disciplines together may have resulted from the impact of the prevailing difficulties in the acute mental health sector. Excessive individual workloads, and the possibility that the timing of the debriefing meeting did not suit the individual professions involved, may both have been influential. The project was not externally funded, and the limited resources available may have been insufficient to maximise positive outcomes in this sort of project.

The ideal of interprofessional learning initiatives promoting more effective team-working among mental health practitioners is not only much vaunted but also open to question (Reeves, 2001; Norman and Peck, 1999). Interested commentators have rightly called for more attention to developing a robust evidence base that addresses the detailed process of training, the maintenance of new skills and practices over time in the clinical environment, and the cost-effectiveness of these initiatives (Gournay and Sandford, 1998; Reeves, 2001). This would require well-resourced and well-designed studies, preferably employing a mixture of quantitative, qualitative and observational methods, which follow up the impact of the training element longitudinally and incorporate service-user focused outcome measures. Ideally, service users would be involved at all stages of the project.

Undoubtedly, single projects of this kind are likely to be expensive to fund. It has been our experience that this is complicated by the requirement of various funding bodies for the training, research and development elements of a project to be disaggregated and costed separately, with funding for each strand sought from different sources. Consequently, bringing together the necessary funding simultaneously for any particular project can prove extremely difficult. Arguably, this state of affairs requires concerted attention from national research and development policymakers if health services are realistically going to address the need to establish evidence-based practices into routine care and organisational systems.

References

Barr H (2000) *Interprofessional Education 1997-2000*. Centre for the Advancement of Interprofessional Education. Report commissioned by the UKCC

Beattie A (1995) War and peace among the health tribes. In: Soothill K, Mackay L, Webb C (Eds). *Interprofessional Relations in Health Care*. Edward Arnold, London: 11–26

Campbell J (1999) Trend spotting: fashions in medical education. *BMJ* **318**: 1272–5

Camsooksai J (2002) The role of the lecturer-practitioner in interprofessional education. *Nurse Educ Today* **22**: 466–75

Carpenter J, Hewstone M (1996) Shared learning for doctors and social workers. *British Journal of Social Work* **26**: 239–57

Clinical Standards Advisory Group Committee on Schizophrenia (1995) *Clinical Standards Advisory Group: Schizophrenia (Volume 1)*. Report of a CSAG committee on schizophrenia. HMSO, London

Cook S (1995) Revisiting interdisciplinary education: one way to build an ark. *N HC Perspect Community* **16**: 5

Cooperrider DL, Srivastva S (1987) Appreciative inquiry in organizational life. In: Woodman R, Pasmore W (Eds). *Research in Organizational Change and Development: Volume 1*. JAI Press, Greenwich, Connecticut: 129–69

Corrigan P, McCracken S (1995) Psychiatric rehabilitation and staff development: educational and organisational models. *Clin Psychol Rev* **15**: 699–719

Corrigan P, McCracken S, Edwards M, Kommana S, Simpatico T (1997) Staff training to improve implementation and impact of behavioural rehabilitation programs. *Psychiatr Serv* **48**: 1336–8

Couchman W (1995) Joint education for mental health teams. *Nurs Stand* **10**(7): 32–4

Department of Health and Social Security (1980) *Organisation and Management Problems of Mental Illness Hospitals: Report of a working group*. HMSO, London

Department of Health (1990) *The Care Programme Approach for People with a Mental Illness Referred to the Specialist Psychiatric Services.* DHSS, London

Department of Health (1994) *Working in Partnership: A collaborative approach to care. Report of the mental health nursing review team* (Butterworth Report). London, HMSO.

Department of Health (1995) *Building Bridges: A guide to arrangements for inter-agency working for the care and protection of severely mentally ill people.* HMSO, London

Department of Health (1996) *The Spectrum of Care: Local services for people with mental health problems.* DoH, London

Department of Health (1997) *Developing Partnerships in Mental Health.* HMSO, London

Department of Health (1998) *Modernising Mental Health Services: Safe, sound and supportive.* DoH, London

Department of Health (1999) *The National Service Framework for Mental Health.* DoH, London

Department of Health (2000) *A Health Service of All the Talents: Developing the NHS workforce.* DoH, London

Department of Health (2001a) *The Expert Patient: A new approach to chronic disease management for the 21st century.* DoH, London

Department of Health (2001b) *The Journey to Recovery — The government's vision for mental health care.* DoH, London

Department of Health, (2002) *Mental Health Policy Implementation Guide: Adult acute inpatient care provision.* DoH, London

DePoy E, Wood C, Miller M (1997) Educating allied health professionals: an interdisciplinary effort. *J Allied Health* **26**: 127–32

Evans S, Carlson R (1992) Nurse/physician collaboration: solving the nursing shortage crisis. *Am J Crit Care* **1**: 25–32

Fadden G (1997) Implementation of family interventions in routine clinical practice following staff training: a major cause for concern. *J Ment Health* **6**(6): 599-612

Frank A, Gunderson J (1990) The role of the therapeutic alliance in the treatment of schizophrenia. *Arch Gen Psychiatry* **47**: 228–36

Finch J (2000) Interprofessional education and teamworking: a view from the education providers. *BMJ* **321**: 1138–40

Glenn S (2002) The way forward. In: Glenn S, Leiba T (Eds). *Multiprofessional Learning for Nurses: Breaking the boundaries.* Palgrave, Basingstoke: 139-47

Gournay K, Sandford T (1998) Training for the workforce. In: Brooker C, Repper J (Eds). *Serious Mental Health Problems in the Community: Policy, practice and research.* Baillière Tindall, London: 291–310

Griffiths L (1997) Accomplishing team: teamwork and categorisation in two community mental health teams. *Sociol Rev* **45**: 59–78

Hammick M (1998) Interprofessional education: concept, theory and application. *J Interprof Care* **12**: 323–32

Harrison L, Kitchens E (1989) Implementing the research facilitator role. *Nurse Educ* **14**(5): 21–6

Headrick L, Wilcock M, Batalden B (1998) Interprofessional working and continuing medical education. *BMJ* **316**: 771–4

Henneman E, Lee J, Cohen J (1995) Collaboration: a concept analysis. *J Adv Nurs* **2**: 103–9

King M, Lee J, Henneman E (1993) A collaborative practice model for critical care. *Am J Crit Care* **2**(6): 444–9

Lancashire S, Haddock G, Tarrier N, Baguley I, Butterworth C, Brooker C (1996) The impact of training community psychiatric nurses to use psychosocial interventions with people who have severe mental health problems. *Psychiatr Serv* **48**: 39–41

Liebling A, Price D, Elliott C (1999) Appreciative inquiry and relationships in prison. *Punishment and Society* **1**(1): 71–98

Mackay L, Soothill K, Webb C (1995) Troubled times: the context for interprofessional collaboration? In: Soothill K, Mackay L, Webb C (Eds). *Interprofessional Relations in Health Care*. Edward Arnold, London: 5–10

Mathias P, Thompson T (1997) Preparation for interprofessional work: trends in education, training and the structure of qualifications in the United Kingdom. In: Ovretveit J, Mathias P, Thompson T (Eds). *Interprofessional Working for Health and Social Care*. Macmillan, Basingstoke: 103–15

McKeown M, Mercer D, Finlayson S (2000) Targeting: the role of training. In: Cotterill L, Barr W (Eds). *Targeting in Mental Health Services*. Ashgate, Aldershot: 219–43

McKeown M, McCann G, Forster J (2002) Psychosocial interventions in institutional settings. In: Harris N, Williams S, Bradshaw S (Eds). *Psychosocial Interventions for People with Schizophrenia*. Palgrave, Basingstoke

Mental Health Act Commission and the Sainsbury Centre (1997). *The National Visit*. The Sainsbury Centre for Mental Health, London

Miller C, Freeman M, Ross N (2001) *Interprofessional Practice in Health and Social Care: Challenging the shared learning agenda*. Arnold, London

Milne D, Westerman C, Hanner S (2002) Can a 'relapse prevention' module facilitate the transfer of training? *Behavioural and Cognitive Psychotherapy* **30**: 361–4

National Health Service Executive (1996) *Education and Training Planning Guidance*. NHSE, London

Norman I, Peck E (1999) Working together in adult community mental health services: an interprofessional dialogue. *J Ment Health* **8**: 217–30

Perkins R, Repper J (1996) *Working Alongside People with Long Term Mental Health Problems*. Chapman & Hall, London

Reeves S (2000) A systematic review of the effects of interprofessional education on staff involved in the care of adults with mental health problems. *J Psychiatric Ment Health Nurs* **8**: 533–42

Reeves S (2001) Community-based interprofessional education for medical, nursing and dental students. *Health and Social Care in the Community* **8**: 269–76

Richardson J, Edwards M (1997) An undergraduate clinical skills laboratory developing interprofessional skills in physical and occupational therapy. *Gerontology and Geriatrics* **17**: 33–43

Rogers A, Pilgrim D, Lacey R (1993) *Experiencing Psychiatry: Users' views of services*. Macmillan in association with MIND Publications, London

Rolls L, Davis E, Coupland K (2002) Improving serious mental illness through interprofessional education. *J Psychiatr Ment Health Nurs* **9**: 317–24

Sainsbury Centre for Mental Health (1997) *Pulling Together: The future roles and training of mental health staff.* Sainsbury Centre for Mental Health, London

Savage L, McKeown M (1997) Towards a new model of practice for a high dependency unit. *Psychiatr Care* **4**: 182–6

Standing Nursing and Midwifery Advisory Committee (SNAMC) (1999) *Mental Health Nursing: Addressing acute concerns.* HMSO, London

Stark S, Stronach I, Warne T (2002) Teamwork in mental health: rhetoric and reality. *J Psychiatr Ment Health Nurs* **9**: 411–18

Van der Horst M, Turpie I, Nelson W (1995) St Joseph's Community Centre model of community-based care team education. *Health and Social Care in the Community* **3**: 33–42

Virgin S, Goodrow B, Duggins B (1996) Scavenger hunt: a community-based learning experience. *Nurse Educ* **21**: 32–4

World Health Organization (1988) *Learning Together to Work Together for Health.* WHO, Geneva

9

Chronic illness: empowering patients for self-care in diabetes

Helen Cooper

Diabetes mellitus is a condition in which the amount of glucose in the blood is abnormally high because of an absolute or relative lack of insulin. There are two main types of diabetes. Both types can be treated and controlled, but not cured.

⌘ **Type 1 diabetes** occurs when there is a severe lack of insulin due to destruction of most or all of the insulin-producing cells, which is usually caused by an autoimmune process. Regular replacement of insulin by injection is essential for the person's survival, alongside a balanced diet and exercise plan to reduce the risks of acute and chronic complications. This type of diabetes usually appears before the age of 40, but may occur at any age and usually has an acute onset. It represents approximately 15–20% of the total diabetes population.

⌘ **Type 2 diabetes** occurs when the body is still producing some insulin but in inadequate amounts, and/or when the insulin that is produced becomes less effective. It is associated with obesity, and in most cases diet and exercise, or diet, exercise and tablets, can improve glucose levels, although insulin is now increasingly being used. This type of diabetes usually appears in people over the age of 40, has a peak age of onset at 60 years, and tends to have a gradual, insidious onset. It is more common in some ethnic groups, particularly Asians.

Both types of diabetes are associated with complications that appear over the longer term. The effects fall into two main groups: microvascular disorders specific to diabetes, which can affect the eyes (diabetic retinopathy), kidneys (nephropathy) and nerves (neuropathy); and an increased risk of large vessel disease such as heart disease, stroke and gangrene.

Clinical and epidemiological data have demonstrated a strong association between the severity of complications and the magnitude and duration of high blood glucose. Two major trials, in particular, confirmed this hypothesis: the Diabetes Control and Complications Trial (DCCT) (DCCT Research Group, 1993) in relation to type 1 diabetes, and the United Kingdom Prospective Diabetes Study (UKPDS, 1998a) in relation to type 2 diabetes. Both showed that an intensive glycaemic control policy, alongside control of lipids, blood pressure and body weight, resulted in significant reductions in the risk of complications. Within this proof, however, lies the enigma of diabetes care: controlling weight, blood glucose, lipids and blood pressure places a huge burden on patients in relation to lifestyle behaviour management. And alongside this, effective drug treatment strategies, combined with surveillance schemes for early detection and treatment of complications, are required.

This highlights the need for a health-promoting approach to diabetes care — one that takes into account the interdependency of patients and healthcare professionals in trying to 'control' the many factors that contribute to both the onset of type 2 diabetes and the development of complications in both types of diabetes.

Prevalence

It is largely the complications associated with diabetes that make it such a major health problem, and one that is escalating with increasing prevalence of the disease. In 1996, it was estimated that type 2 diabetes affected 11 million people worldwide; by the year 2010 it is estimated that more than 215 million individuals will be affected (Audit Commission, 2000). Furthermore, it is hypothesised that half of diabetes cases remain undiagnosed. Zimmet and Lefebvre (1996) suggest that the most important factors contributing to such growth are ageing, urbanisation (predominantly in developing countries), sedentary lifestyle and increasing prevalence of obesity. In England and Wales alone, nearly half the population are overweight (body mass index >25), and 20%, or 11 million people, are obese (body mass index >30) (Barth, 2002). In addition, in 1999, the World Health Organization (WHO) revised the diagnosis and classification of diabetes, resulting in a lowered threshold for diagnosis (WHO, 1999). This in itself has impacted on the prevalence of diabetes worldwide and, correspondingly, the demands on heath service resources.

To meet such demands, the Government in the UK has focused on integrated teamwork and developing patient expertise to promote empowerment (Department of Health [DoH], 2001a). This philosophy is based on a simple expedient, namely that the knowledge and experience held by patients is an untapped resource. It is hypothesised that the utilisation of such expertise within the diabetes team will benefit the quality of patients' care and ultimately their quality of life. Such a shift of emphasis requires recognition of the active role that patients and their carers need to adopt. It reinforces the view that the responsibility for chronic disease management ultimately resides with the patient, and that care for chronic disease is a completely different social activity from care for acute illness. This highlights the need for a change in the way that health professionals approach patient care, shifting the emphasis towards the role of educator, facilitator and supporter.

From a purely historical perspective, team-working and patient empowerment in diabetes care is not new. As long ago as 1932, RD Lawrence, one of the founders of the patients' charity 'Diabetes UK' wrote:

'In the successful treatment of diabetes, the patient, the nurse, the practitioner and the specialist are often partners working together to establish the patient's health. In the long run, the most important part, the melody, is played by the patient, and the accompaniment may be almost unheard.'

(Lawrence, 1932)

Perhaps the most telling part of his philosophy is that he too had diabetes.

This chapter reviews current patterns of care and the importance of self-management in diabetes mellitus. Promotion of patient empowerment is debated in the context of patient education, with particular focus on the theoretical framework underpinning practice and the need for a team approach to care. It includes a discussion of the potential changes required to enhance and maintain the effects of patient empowerment, and the implications of this for interprofessional healthcare education. An example of how such recommendations have been implemented is provided, and lessons learnt from this experience are discussed.

Patterns of care

Patterns of care for people with diabetes have been changing over the last 20 years. In the past, the hospital was seen as the main facilitator of care. More recently, shared care has emerged as it became evident that there were too many patients for hospitals to be the sole provide of care. The role of primary care has therefore steadily increased, particularly in relation to management of type 2 diabetes. This practice has reflected an overall strategic vision for health services in which secondary care exists to support and to respond to the agenda of primary care (DoH, 1997). The main focus is on integration of all available resources both within the NHS and without. This demands the development of sophisticated patterns of inter-agency and interprofessional working.

To achieve such patterns of care, recent approaches have adopted a public health stance. This approach began in 1990 with publication of the St Vincent Declaration – the first document to set targets for the prevention of complications associated with diabetes (WHO [Europe] and International Diabetes Federation [Europe], 1990). The Declaration was an agreement of all European countries, under the auspices of the WHO and the International Diabetes Federation (IDF), to improve care for people with diabetes. It evolved from the work of the WHO on health promotion, and specifically refers to the document *Targets for Health for All* (WHO, 1985) as having directed its evolution.

It formulated a series of recommendations, which, in the UK, were translated as a need to establish a new role for patients — one in which self-management and partnerships play a lead part. This approach leant itself to the principles of patient empowerment and was reinforced by publication of National Service Frameworks (NSF) for Diabetes in England (DoH 2001b), and similar guidance in Wales (National Assembly for Wales, 2001), Northern Ireland (DoH Social Services and Public Safety for Northern Ireland, 2000) and Scotland (SIGN, 2001) which describe standards for diabetes care and call for collaboration between all involved, including the patient, as an empowered force. Standard 3 in the English Framework document, for example, refers to empowering people with diabetes to:

> '... enhance their personal control over the day-to-day management of their diabetes in a way that enables them to experience the best possible quality of life.'

The strategy for health and wellbeing in Northern Ireland recognises that:

> '... the impact of diabetes on patients' daily lives and the chances of complications can be reduced through the provision of well-organised integrated care.'

Patient self-management is therefore seen as the key to good diabetes care, and patient education to promote such empowered behaviour should be at the heart of any service.

Empowerment and the diabetes patient

Various researchers have shown that empowerment encourages individuals with diabetes to develop their own strategies for self-management (Hurley and Shea, 1992; Kavanagh et al 1993; Anderson, 1995). Others have found that such an approach is limited by the need for an organisational culture that supports the devolution of power to the individual patient (Rayman and Ellison, 1998; Thorne et al, 2000). However, Skinner and Cradock (2000) conducted a narrative review of patient empowerment and diabetes literature and found that its value could only be argued for on philosophical grounds because, at that time, no published empirical studies existed that had rigorously tested its application.

Alongside this, an Audit Commission Report (2000) in the UK exposed severe deficits in understanding of the disease among people who have diabetes, with two-thirds of patients saying they had received no education or support within the previous 12 months. In line with this finding, the Commission found that arrangements for patient education were variable across the trusts surveyed, with less than half the hospitals having comprehensive programmes for patient education and only one hospital evaluating the education that patients received. The report's recommendations reinforced the need for an evidence base for patient education to provide guidance to the multidisciplinary team.

Lessons from patient education research

The evidence base for diabetes patient education includes both traditional literature reviews that embody the subjective opinions of experts, and meta-analyses of the published literature. Posavac (1980), Mazzuca (1982) and Mullen *et al* (1985) measured the effect of education using meta-analysis for people with a range of diseases that included diabetes. Various papers have discussed the evidence for rethinking the models of diabetes patient education, making recommendations based on the literature (Assal *et al* ,1985; Glasgow, 1995; Rayman and Ellison, 1998).

A systematic review of the literature on diabetes patient education was funded by Diabetes UK in 1999 (Griffin *et al*, 1998). The unpublished report included a narrative survey of seven meta-analyses of patient education, and summarised 57 published controlled trials with a focus on methodological strengths and weaknesses. It found that research into diabetes education had demonstrated desirable outcomes in the short term, but failed to demonstrate whether these effects were sustained over the longer term. A subsequent report published by Diabetes UK recommended that patient education should be a planned lifelong process, starting at the point of diagnosis and remaining as an essential component of diabetes care (Naqib, http://www.diabetes. org.uk/ education/edreport.doc).

These results were confirmed in a second review of patient education for a broad range of chronic diseases that have lifestyle behaviour change as part of their treatment programmes. This behavioural component was taken as the common link between diabetes, hypertension, hyperlipidaemia, coronary heart disease and arthritis (Cooper *et al*, 2001). A narrative and critical review of twelve meta-analyses of patient education for these diseases showed that, while a great deal of research has been conducted, its methodological rigour was questionable and there were insufficient rigorous data to judge the effects of patient education. Where randomised controlled trials (RCTs) had been conducted, the effect size was usually small and was only known for six months of follow-up. In addition, the educational interventions tested were poorly described and failed to adhere to theoretical models. The meta-analyses could not therefore provide a clear answer to the question of what types of educational interventions produce maximum benefits for patients.

The information that could be discerned showed that practitioners need to use theory-based teaching strategies that include behaviour change tactics that affect feelings and attitudes towards a disease and its treatment. Such an approach relies upon exploration of the theories associated with health protective behaviours, alongside the theories associated with educational strategies employed to effect these behaviours. These theories provide a generic tool for implementing patient education. They provide a framework of variables that can be used to direct practice (how to do it), intervention goals (what to achieve), and possible explanations for any outcomes of an intervention. An appreciation of these theories can therefore provide guidance on how to tailor interventions to suit patients' needs so that patients can achieve what is appropriate for them at any particular time in their illness career. This is a fundamental principle of empowerment and has implications for interprofessional training.

Healthcare education

The Diabetes NSF focuses on patient empowerment and integrated team-working. The realisation of such a vision, however, depends upon formal preparation for this way of working. Professional education, as it currently stands, does not equip practitioners with these skills. It is therefore necessary to add such learning into professional education at both undergraduate and postgraduate levels. The topic represents a common learning module for all health and social care professionals under the umbrella of health promotion, which has been identified by higher education's Quality Assurance Agency (QAA) as one of the foundations of professional practice. The development and implementation of such a module would provide the fit between curricula and NSF programmes. It would also begin the cultural shift that is needed to provide interprofessional teams with the skills and abilities to support patients in their lifelong task of maintaining their own health.

This reflects a policy of developing practitioners who are fit for purpose, but anxieties still exist about the theory–practice gap at qualification (Rafferty, 1992). To overcome such barriers, there is a need to involve clinically based staff. Students then have role models at the 'sharp end' of health care on whom to align their attitudes, skills, knowledge and behaviour. In this way they are more likely to be convinced of the relevance of what they are learning to the practice of their discipline of health care. In addition, teaching methods need to exemplify good practice, reflecting those that can be used with patients. These should follow general educational principles that have been defined by several writers, including Knowles (1973) on adult learning, Kolb (1984) on experiential learning, and Schon (1987) on reflective practice. In a dynamic healthcare environment, practitioners need to become self-directed, critical thinkers and reflective practitioners. As Rawnsley (1990) stated:

> *'When living the reality of their practice, [health professionals] need ways through which they can connect the conceptual concerns of [their] discipline with the raw data of experience.'*

Learning through reflection therefore involves attempting to resolve the contradictions between what professionals currently do and what is desirable practice. As for patients, professional education must aim to affect knowledge, skills, attitudes and eventually behaviour. This demonstrates the overlap between both parties in relation to adult experiential learning (*Table 9.1*).

Table 9.1: General educational principles to guide adult learning

Adult learners should:

⌘ Be involved in all aspects of learning

⌘ Base their learning on previous experiences

⌘ Set their own learning objectives

⌘ Relate their learning to real-life problems

⌘ Reflect on their learning experiences

⌘ Develop new ideas and put them into practice

⌘ Be involved in evaluating their learning

⌘ Give and receive feedback on their progress

⌘ Be provided with a conducive learning environment (both physical and emotional)

Goals of healthcare education

Healthcare professionals can only buy into the empowerment model of healthcare if they accept its underlying goals. Without this understanding, misconceptions about what shared decision-making in health care involves will continue. The Government's agenda is to develop patient expertise (DoH, 2001a), and within this there is an emphasis upon health professionals working in partnerships with patients and involving them in decision-making about their own treatment and self-care. These goals are presented as compatible, and their mutual implementation is presumed to lead to a 'first-class service' (DoH, 1998). Without interprofessional learning around a common curriculum, there is a potential for conflict as each professional group gains differing understandings of what empowerment really means. Atkinson (1981) notes that medical expertise is developed not simply through the possession of relevant knowledge, but is based on experiential learning in the clinical setting. It is this expertise that underpins the professional nature of medicine.

The power relations between patients and health professionals are therefore challenged when patients also develop relevant knowledge, which, together with their experiential learning, compromise their usual passive role. It is this change in the professional–patient relationship that underpins acceptance of patient empowerment by both patients and professionals alike and reinforces the need for interdisciplinary learning around a common health promotion curriculum.

Common learning modules

The Centre for Advancement of Interprofessional Education (CAIPE) defines multiprofessional education as:

> '… *a learning process in which people from different professional backgrounds learn together. The content of the learning is therefore common*'

and interprofessional education (IPE) as:

> '… *a learning process in which different professionals learn from, and about each other, in order to develop collaborative practice.*'
> (CAIPE; http://www.caipe.org.uk/)

Common learning modules are therefore oriented towards multiprofessional education. They aim to standardise specific areas of health and social care education programmes and therefore need to be designed from an interdisciplinary perspective. To do this, there is a need to develop working relationships between different professional groups. Field and Schuller (1997) argue that it is the nature of such relationships that purport to make up a learning society. Thus, measures of success include how far people in different departments actually share information, and how far they are able to trust others to pursue common goals. Such an interdisciplinary team approach implies that the more information and values are shared, the more effective the system will be in encouraging adults (patients and professionals) to learn. This is key to developing a strategy for patient care teams in chronic disease management. Above all, it means thinking about learning not just as something that draws on the abilities of individuals, but as something that requires, develops and also makes use of relationships.

Implementing recommendations into practice

One of the cornerstones of health care to support active patient participation is continuity of care between different professional groups. This was clearly highlighted in my own research on the effects of an empowering education programme aimed at people with type 2 diabetes. The trial undertook to put recommendations into practice by overcoming the gaps identified in reviews of patient education research. It addressed the following questions:
Would participation in a theoretically constructed educational programme:

- have an impact upon patients' illness beliefs?
- lead to changes in self-care behaviours?
- have an impact upon blood glucose control?

These questions were addressed using both quantitative (randomised controlled wait list trial) and qualitative (focus group interviews) research methods over a short (six months) and long (twelve months) period. A total of eighty-nine people with type 2 diabetes took part. The quantitative methods focused on exploring outcomes in relation to self-care behaviours (diet, exercise, self-monitoring), physiological effects (blood glucose levels, HbA_{1c}, weight and drug treatment changes) and psychological outcomes (attitudes and personal models of diabetes). Qualitative methods explored patients' perceptions of the educational intervention and its effects (Cooper *et al*, 2002).

Preparing for the trial

The intervention used in the trial was based on the Health Education Authority's 'Look After Yourself' (LAY) programme. Central to its philosophy was an empowerment approach to health education, and as such it was based on the premise that the acquisition of knowledge is not sufficient to equip individuals for self-directed action. It stressed that knowledge needed to be combined with motivation and a range of skills in order to promote action. The course comprised three parts, as outlined in *Table 9.2*.

The training course to teach LAY was a generic course aimed at both the public and health professionals. It provided a unique way of bringing different professional groups and patients together to learn about how people change and the practical skills of change management. It aimed to enable tutors to increase their understanding of how adults learn in groups and to develop their group management skills. They were also trained to teach the exercise and relaxation programme associated with the course.

Table 9.2: Structure of the 'Look After Yourself' (LAY) course

Component	Approach
Physical activity and exercise	A safe, effective personalised programme designed for all individuals, whatever their capabilities and starting levels of fitness. Individuals are encouraged to choose activities and exercises that best meet their needs. It is non-competitive and progress is monitored using pulse rates, perceived exertion and personal record cards.
Relaxation	A neuromuscular tension control programme which offers individuals the opportunity to develop relaxation skills that can be applied to everyday situations.
Health topics	Exploration of lifestyle issues and their links with health in the context of individuals' needs, circumstances and priorities; this includes examination of external factors as well as individual behaviour.

The diabetes course was constructed using the basic LAY programme as its template. It was structured to cover the cardiovascular risk factors associated with type 2 diabetes over an eight-week period (*Table 9.3*). It included both a teaching package for patients and a training package for health professionals who had completed the LAY course. Its primary aim was to reduce the risks of complications of the disease through the development of an empowered approach to self-care.

It utilised a variety of teaching strategies designed to improve psychological wellbeing and promote consciousness-raising and self-efficacy. These strategies included group discussion, role-playing, goal setting, relaxation and practice of skills. Learning from each other was also encouraged by inviting individuals to interact with other group members to seek information, to confirm or disprove their beliefs about diabetes, and to fill in gaps in their knowledge. In this way, individuals within the group were recognised as having personal expertise in the management of their diabetes, while group processes were used to encourage changes in beliefs and values about diabetes. As the groups became more established, members were encouraged to challenge their own and others' assumptions and to integrate their new-found knowledge, skills and attitudes into their own life situation.

The relaxation component was seen as incremental to other parts of the course that deal with participants' feelings about being diagnosed with diabetes and fears of complications associated with the disease. In this way, the diabetes course addressed a 'grey area' of diabetes, which education programmes have tended not to address in the past (Zettler *et al*, 1995). Participants were encouraged to share their feelings, and the ways they have coped, with group members.

Table 9.3: Diabetes patient training programme: health topics

Content	Week 1	Weeks 2 & 3	Week 4	Weeks 5 & 6	Week 7	Week 8
Introduction to the course and other	√					
Overview of diabetes self-management	√	√	√	√	√	√
Nutrition		√	√			
Physical activity and exercise			√			
Exploration of feelings about having diabetes				√		
Making lifestyle changes		√	√	√	√	
Blood glucose self-monitoring		√	√	√	√	
Screening					√	
Reducing the risks of complications			√	√	√	√
Making treatment decisions			√	√	√	√
Informing the healthcare team					√	√
Working with healthcare professionals						√
Making an action plan	√	√		√	√	√

Alongside this, interactive teaching aids, called 'diabetes boxes', were specifically designed for the course by the researcher, working in liaison with a group of artists from a registered charity (Cooper and Jones, 2002). Each box is a three-dimensional tailor-made cube with a specific theme: 'Living with diabetes', 'Changing behaviour' and 'Preventing complications'. The boxes were employed to stimulate group discussion, to help people develop an understanding of the biological and psychological concepts relating to diabetes, and to help people articulate their feelings about having the disease.

Results

The results demonstrated significant changes in HbA$_{1c}$ ($P=0.005$) at six months, but not at twelve months ($P=0.08$). Significant improvements in participants' psychological attitudes towards diabetes were noted at six months ($P=0.04$) and twelve months ($P=0.01$). No significant changes in self-monitoring behaviours were detected at six months, but changes were highly significant at twelve months ($P=0.002$). Positive improvements in diet and exercise behaviour were also noted, but these did not reach significance.

The focus group data showed that the intervention moved participants towards self-care and feelings of personal control over their disease. It helped participants enter the behaviour change cycle, but the relationship with healthcare professionals was critical to the long-term results of this outcome. Kieffer (1984) states that empowerment involves relationships with others because it is '…nurtured by the effects of collaborative efforts'. It is clear from this statement that empowerment is about the relationship between individuals and their environment; this relationship is reciprocal and can serve to affect, positively and negatively, health outcomes. The relationships with the tutors, and with others who have diabetes, had a positive effect, which the majority of participants were able to maintain over the trial period. Where social and/or environmental factors conspired against participants, some of these positive effects were not maintained. In particular, participants spoke about the delimiting effects of health professionals who employ a biomedical approach to their illness, and the negative effects of lack of support at home. Such findings emphasise the importance of healthcare professionals moving towards a more social paradigm of care if the short-term benefits of patient education are to be maintained.

The trial therefore showed that patient education can empower individuals with diabetes to develop their own strategies for self-management. It highlighted that patient education is a long-term process and that all members of the diabetes team have a part to play. This in turn emphasises the need for an interdisciplinary approach to patient education – one in which all members of a team work from a similar understanding of education – and the need to value patients' expertise and to work in partnership with patients.

Lessons learnt

What differentiated this research from other educational studies is the work undertaken before its commencement. Development and piloting of the course over a four-year period involved multidisciplinary collaborative work between a range of health professionals, health educators, artists, patients and researchers. In addition, lessons learnt from a detailed examination of patient education research were utilised to ensure a rigorous approach to the design of the research study. In implementing the trial, a number of valuable lessons were learnt. These included:

• the need for an open communication policy
• the need to value everyone's contribution
• recognition and utilisation of patients' and professionals' experience
• training programmes that follow the principles of adult education, with their focus on experiential learning
• confidence to consult and involve people outside the NHS
• exploration of creative ways of learning
• patient feedback to strengthen the perceived value of the intervention
• embracing opportunities when they arise.

The trial results highlighted a number of issues that need to be addressed, including:

⌘ Recognition of the value of ongoing education by everyone involved in diabetes care, including the patient.
⌘ Development of an integrated team approach to patient education, promoted through shared education and training and through locally agreed guidelines and protocols.
⌘ The need to build imaginative networks that integrate all available resources for patient education.

Conclusions

Over the past few years, patient education has been recognised at clinical, management and governmental levels as key to improving outcomes for people with diabetes. Various reports, however, have highlighted shortfalls in the provision of such education. They have found that it is interpreted and delivered in different ways, and usually offered on an ad-hoc basis. As a result, diabetes education is regarded as an optional service to the patient, and is frequently haphazard and fragmented. This has affected beliefs about the value of education and contributed to a lack of understanding about how it can be effectively integrated into patient care.

Alongside this, patient education is delivered by a variety of providers. This does not, in itself, constitute team care. A functional team is characterised by regular communication among its members and the pursuit of common and agreed goals. As a member of this team, the person with diabetes should be provided with sufficient information to be fully involved in his or her own care plan. This highlights the importance of collaborative education and training for all, including the patient. The purpose of this chapter has been to demonstrate the need for such an educational policy. This has been done by:

- reviewing the increasing public health burden of diabetes
- looking at patterns of care with a focus on the NSF
- discussing patient empowerment
- reviewing a trial of an empowering educational intervention.

Taken together, this evidence supports the need for IPE at all levels of training.

References

Anderson RM (1995) Patient empowerment and the traditional medical model: a case of irreconcilable differences? *Diabetes Care* **18**: 4112–15

Assal JP, Muhlhauser I, Pernet A, Gfeller R, Jorgens V, Berger M (1985) Patient education as the basis for diabetes care in clinical practice and research. *Diabetologia* **28**: 602–13

Atkinson P (1981) *The Clinical Experience: The construction and reconstruction of medical reality*. Gower, Guilford: 110–14

Audit Commission (2000) *Testing Times. A review of diabetes services in England and Wales*. The Audit Commission for local authorities and the National Health Service in England and Wales, London

Barth JH (2002) What should we do about the obesity epidemic? *Practical Diabetes International* **19**: 119–22

Cooper H, Jones A (2002) Connecting art to healthcare education: evaluation of a project with ethnic minority groups in Liverpool. *Diabet Med* **19** (Suppl 2): A90, 23

Cooper H, Booth K, Fear S, Gill G (2001) Lessons from chronic disease patient education. *Patient Education and Counselling* **44**: 107–17

Cooper H, Booth K, Gill G (2002) Diabetes education: the patient's perspective. *Journal of Diabetes Nursing* **6**(3): 91-5

Department of Health (1997) *The New NHS: Modern, dependable*. NHS White Paper. HMSO, London

Department of Health (1998) *Our Healthier Nation*. HMSO, London

Department of Health (2001a) *The Expert Patient. A new approach to chronic disease management for the 21st century*. HMSO, London

Department of Health (2001b) *National Service Framework for Diabetes. Standards document*. DoH, London

Department of Health, Social Services and Public Safety (DHSSPS) for Northern Ireland (2000) *Investing for Health – Consultation paper*. DHSSPS, Belfast

Diabetes Control and Complications Trial Research Group (1993) The effect of intensive treatment of diabetes on the development and progression of long-term complications in insulin-dependent diabetes mellitus *N Engl J Med* **329**: 977–86

Field J, Schuller T (1997) Norms, networks ands trust. *Adults Learning* **November**: 17–18

Glasgow R (1995) A practical working model of diabetes management and education. *Diabetes Care* **18**: 117-26

Griffin S, Kinmouth AL, Skinner C, Kelly J (1998) *Educational and psychosocial interventions for adults with diabetes*. Report for the British Diabetic Association

Hurley AC, Shea, CA (1992) Self-efficacy: strategy for enhancing diabetes self-care. *Diabetes Educ* **18**: 146–50

Kavanagh DJ, Gooley S, Wilson PH (1993) Prediction of adherence and control in diabetes. *J Behav Med* **16**: 509–22

Kieffer C (1984) Citizen empowerment: a developmental perspective. *Prev Hum Serv* **3**: 9–36

Knowles MS (1973) *The Adult Learner: A neglected species*. Gulf Publishing Company, Houston, Texas

Kolb DA (1984) *Experiential Learning: Experience as the source of learning and development*. Prentice Hall, Englewood Cliffs, New Jersey

Lawrence RD (1932) *The Diabetic ABC*. HK Lewis, London

Mazzuca SA (1982) Does patient education in chronic disease have therapeutic value? *Journal of Chronic Disability* **35**: 521–9

Mullen PD, Green LW, Persinger GS (1985) Clinical trials of patient education for chronic conditions: a comparative meta-analysis of intervention types. *Prev Med* **14**: 753–81

National Assembly for Wales (2001) The people's NHS: Public and patient involvement. In: *Improving Health in Wales: A plan for the NHS and its partners*. National Assembly for Wales, Cardiff

Naqib J. *Patient Education for Effective Diabetes Self-management. Report, recommendations and examples of good practice*. Published on: http://www.diabetes.org.uk/education/ edreport.doc. Accessed March 2004

Posavac EJ (1980) Evaluations of patient education programs. *Eval Health Prof* **3**: 47–62

Rafferty D (1992) Implications of the theory-practice gap for project 2000 students. *Br J Nurs* **1**: 507–13

Rawnsley M (1990) Of human bonding: the context of nursing as caring. *Advanced Nursing Science* **13**: 41–8

Rayman KM, Ellison GC (1998) When management works: an organisational culture that facilitates learning to self-manage Type 2 diabetes. *Diabetes Educ* **24**: 612–17

Schon DA (1987) *Educating the Reflective Practitioner*. Jossey-Bass, San Francisco

SIGN (Scottish Intercollegiate Guidelines Network) (2001) *Management of Diabetes*. SIGN, Edinburgh

Skinner TC, Cradock S (2000) Empowerment: what about the evidence? *Practical Diabetes International* **17**: 91–5

Thorne SE, Nyhlin KT, Paterson BL (2000) Attitudes toward patient expertise in chronic illness. *Int J Nurs Stud* **37**: 303–11

UK Prospective Diabetes Study (UKPDS) Group (1998) Intensive blood glucose control with sulphonylureas or insulin compared with conventional treatment and risk of complications in patients with type 2 diabetes (UKPDS 33). *Lancet* **352**: 837–53

World Health Organization (1985) *Targets for Health for All*. WHO, Geneva

World Health Organization (Europe) and International Diabetes Federation (Europe) (1990) Diabetes care and research in Europe: The St Vincent Declaration. *Diabet Med* **7**: 360

World Health Organization (1999) *Definition, Diagnosis and Classification of Diabetes Mellitus and its Complications. Report of the WHO Collaboration*. WHO, Geneva

Zettler A, Duran G, Waadt S, Herschbach P, Struan F (1995) Coping with fear of complications in diabetes mellitus: a model clinical program. *Psychother Psychosoms* **64**: 178–84

Zimmet P, Lefebvre P (1996) The global NIDDM pandemic: treating the disease and ignoring the symptoms. *Diabetologia* **39**: 1247–8

10

Learning disabilities: building team-working for the future

Tim Riding

The face of learning disability services has changed beyond recognition since the publication of *Better Services for the Mentally Handicapped* (Department of Health [DoH], 1971). Following the subsequent shift from long-stay hospital care to community-based provision, the ideal of ordinary, valued and socially inclusive lifestyles was given a renewed emphasis with the unveiling of the Government's ambitious White Paper *Valuing People: A new strategy for learning disability for the 21st century* (DoH, 2001). A central theme of the new strategy is that people with learning disabilities should use mainstream services wherever possible, and specialist services only where necessary. Furthermore, where the use of specialist services is required, there should be a re-focusing of their expertise to enhance the competence and capacity of local services.

This challenge brings with it a range of opportunities for interprofessional education (IPE) with colleagues in mental health services, primary healthcare teams, social services and the independent sector. This chapter therefore explores the key issues to be addressed if the vision set out in *Valuing People* is to become a reality. Initially, the current policy context for learning disability services will be appraised, and will lead into a discussion of the concept of health in people with learning disabilities. The challenges of, and opportunities for, IPE that arise will be highlighted, supported by proposals of how the agenda can be taken forward. The chapter will conclude with specific examples of how the issues are already being addressed on a practical level in some areas.

Policy context

In 1995, following a DoH-commissioned report into the role of the learning disability nurse (Kay *et al*, 1995), a supplementary guide promoting collaboration between primary and specialist health services was published (DoH, 1995). It acknowledged that, in addition to the health problems experienced by the general population, people with learning disabilities were more likely to suffer from a range of associated conditions, including epilepsy, hearing and visual impairments, communication problems, obesity, and cardiovascular and gastrointestinal abnormalities. Some three years later, following recognition that access to good quality health services was still not the norm for the majority of people with learning disabilities, a further guide *Signposts for Success in Commissioning and Providing Health Services for People with Learning Disabilities* was issued, once again aiming to promote good practice in the commissioning and provision of relevant health services (NHS Executive, 1998).

Signposts for Success promoted the view that the health needs of people with learning disabilities had not changed, but the way their needs are met had. Whereas 'mental handicap' hospitals had once provided the main source of health care, following the closure of the majority of such hospitals, most people with learning disabilities now lived in the community and were hence expected to access mainstream primary care, community and hospital services. Nonetheless, it was also recognised that, despite a range of policy initiatives, uptake of services was considerably lower than expected, and it was suggested that the benefits of dispersed community services carried an associated risk of failure to identify and subsequently address health needs (NHS Executive, 1998).

The Social Services Inspectorate report *Moving into the Mainstream* (Social Services Inspectorate, 1998) confirmed many of these fears. Access to primary and community health services was found to be problematic, especially for those with additional sensory impairments, and admissions to acute hospitals were characterised by problems arising from the additional 'social care' needs of people with learning disabilities. Such concerns were further echoed through the policy impact study *Facing the Facts*, carried out in 1998/99 across 24 local authority areas in England (DoH, 1999). Significant problems were once again reported regarding the development of, and access to, primary, specialist and continuing healthcare services, with the difficulties exacerbated for those with complex or additional physical or mental health needs. Three underlying problems were identified:

⌘ The relationship between the NHS and local authorities in relation to the provision of continuing care was unclear, with only half having agreed joint eligibility criteria.

⌘ There was considerable evidence of health professionals being 'out of tune' with the experience of people with learning disabilities within the healthcare system.

⌘ The fragmentation of service systems had resulted in huge variability of service both within and across local authority areas.

The need for development and implementation of policies and procedures was identified, together with a comprehensive training strategy. It was suggested that primary care groups, in the strategic commissioning of learning disability services, would lead the debate as to how community learning disability teams could influence other forms of health service provision (DoH, 1999).

In response, the NHS Executive produced further good practice guidance emphasising the responsibility of primary healthcare teams in meeting the health needs of people with learning disabilities. *Once a Day* (NHS Executive, 1999) highlighted the need for such teams to develop strong links with specialist teams for people with learning disabilities, promoting partnership working with other health and local authority services. The guidance was designed to stimulate primary healthcare services to become more accessible and responsive to people with learning disabilities, and to identify areas in which involvement of the local specialist services may be helpful:

> *'We are not asking primary healthcare staff to develop new technical or specialist skills. But they will need to ensure that their services are flexible and capable of meeting the needs of every person registered with their practice. Meeting the needs of a person with a learning disability should become routine good practice rather than be seen as a problem to be overcome.'*
>
> (Hutton, 1999a: 1)

Some of the difficulties experienced in meeting the *physical* healthcare needs of people with learning disabilities were mirrored in the provision of *mental* health services. Following the long-stay hospital closure programme, people with learning disabilities are increasingly likely to be admitted to a general adult psychiatric ward, particularly during a first psychotic episode (Doody, 2001). Therefore, citing the work of the Royal College of Psychiatrists (1996), who highlighted the difficulties of enabling people with learning disabilities to use ordinary mental health services, Chaplin and Flynn (2000: 128) propose two overriding principles:

> *'Joint working between general and specialist psychiatrist, and the use of generic or general psychiatric facilities where appropriate.'*

However, despite the succession of service reviews and resultant policy initiatives and good practice guidance, there was little evidence of positive change, as people with learning disabilities continued to experience difficulties across the spectrum of primary and secondary care. The much-heralded National Service Frameworks (NSFs) were seen by many as the catalyst that would surmount many of the problems, although there was both confusion and dismay as to why learning disabilities was merely to have a 'strategy' (Hutton, 1999b) instead. In reality, the fact that there was to be no specific NSF for people with learning disabilities implied that, by default, each and every NSF applied equally to people with learning disabilities and the general population. Nevertheless, there was great anticipation when it was at last announced that the learning disability strategy was in fact to be afforded White Paper status (Hutton, 2000).

Valuing People: A new strategy for learning disability for the 21st century (DoH, 2001) was eventually presented to Parliament in March 2001, and set out a new vision underpinned by the four key principles of rights, independence, choice and inclusion. National objectives for learning disability services were set, supported by new targets and performance indicators. With regard to improving health, a number of fundamental challenges were identified, including:

⌘ All people with a learning disability should be registered with a GP by June 2004.

⌘ Health facilitators would be identified by Spring 2003 and the opportunity for health action plans offered to all people with a learning disability by June 2005.

⌘ All mainstream hospital services were to be made available to people with learning disabilities.

⌘ The benefits of the NSF for Mental Health should be realised by people with learning disabilities also.

In pursuit of these aims, it was acknowledged that the role of the specialist learning disability teams had to change to facilitate the work of mainstream services. It was proposed that specialist staff should give less time to direct interventions and more to developing capability within local services to support those with complex needs. The additional complementary roles advocated are outlined in *Table 10.1*. Clearly, there was a need for much greater emphasis on partnership working with the whole range of services and agencies involved in delivering care and treatment to people with learning disabilities, although, in the absence of robust health needs assessments, the specific needs of local populations remained unclear. So, what exactly are the health problems likely to be experienced by people with learning disabilities?

Meeting the health needs of people with a learning disability

A recent review of the contribution of all nurses to the care and support of people with learning disabilities, commissioned by the Scottish Executive, identified people with learning disabilities as having three broad categories of health need:

● everyday health needs
● health needs resulting from a learning disability
● complex health needs.

Everyday health needs are seen as those experienced by the general population, for whom the GP is often regarded as the 'gatekeeper' to primary and secondary care, health education and promotion, and a range of preventive strategies, including routine health checks and screening programmes (Scottish Executive Health Department, 2002). Therefore, if people with learning disabilities are to have their everyday needs met through mainstream services, there is a need for at least a basic understanding of learning disability across the whole spectrum of health care.

Roberts (2002) proposes six generic competencies required by health professionals lacking a learning disability qualification:

- an ability to recognise, in any clinical setting, someone with a learning disability
- effective communication skills
- an ability to identify unmet health needs
- an appreciation that behaviour often masks underlying health needs
- an appreciation of the relationship between disability and health
- an ability to work in partnership with families, carers and specialist colleagues.

In attaining these competencies, staff in primary care teams and hospital settings will undoubtedly be better placed to meet everyday health needs. However, it is argued that a focus on everyday needs alone may result in other basic health needs — those specifically associated with learning disabilities — not being identified (Turner and Moss, 1996). The focus must therefore be broadened to take account of those additional health needs likely to be experienced.

Table 10.1: Complementary roles for specialist services

In addition to their clinical and therapeutic roles, specialist staff should take on the following complementary tasks:

⌘ A health promotion role — working closely with the local health promotion team.

⌘ A health facilitation role — working with primary care teams, community health professionals and staff involved in delivering secondary health care.

⌘ A teaching role – to enable a wide range of staff, including those who work in social services and the independent sector, to become more familiar with how to support people with learning disabilities to have their health needs met.

⌘ A service development role — contributing their knowledge of health issues to planning processes.

Reproduced from *Valuing People* (DoH, 2001, p. 69)

There is overwhelming evidence to suggest that people with learning disabilities are likely to experience a much greater range of health needs, many of which are frequently unmet (Howells, 1986; Barker and Howells, 1990; Meehan *et al,* 1995; Hunt *et al,* 2001). Indeed, it is argued that, at any point in time, approximately 40% of adults with a learning disability will have an additional mental health need and as many as 70% will have an additional physical health need (Cooper, 1997; Cooper and Bailey, 2001). Additional health needs are defined as those arising directly from the underlying cause of the learning disability, and those that result from the experience of disability (Matthews *et al,* 2002; Scottish Executive Health Department, 2002).

To clarify, a person with Down's syndrome is more likely to experience congenital heart defects and cataracts, and is at greater risk of developing thyroid dysfunction, depression and dementia (ie. directly related to the underlying cause) (Scottish Executive Health Department, 2002). A recent study undertaken in people with learning disabilities also revealed, among other things, that two-thirds of the sample were overweight, many of whom experienced associated mobility problems. This was attributed, at least in part, to poor dietary habits coexisting with a lack of exercise (i.e. the experience of disability) (Matthews *et al,* 2002). A range of biological, psychological and social factors have also been cited in the aetiology of mental health problems in this client group, including: brain damage and sensory impairment; cognitive and emotional responses to life events such as bereavement; the increased risk of abuse; and a lack of meaningful relationships and activities (Hardy and Bouras, 2002).

A more proactive approach, involving a range of services and professionals, is hence required to prevent and minimise the effects of additional health needs, for example, annual blood-testing to detect early hypothyroidism in people with Down's syndrome (Scottish Executive Health Department, 2002), or training in the use of the Psychiatric Assessment Schedule for Adults with Developmental Disabilities (PAS-ADD) checklist (Moss *et al,* 1998) for direct care workers to enable them to identify the early onset of mental health problems. Clearly, there is a need for greater IPE if such an approach is to be achieved. For example, primary care teams must be able to recognise the presence of a learning disability in order to identify those people on their practice lists requiring additional screening or intervention (Roberts, 2002). Similarly, learning disability practitioners must develop and maintain an awareness of associated health needs in order to facilitate access to primary care for their clients, and subsequently support their primary care colleagues (DoH, 2001).

However, many people with learning disabilities also have health needs that require additional specialist support above and beyond that provided by mainstream services. The term 'complex needs' has been coined to describe situations whereby everyday health needs coexist alongside additional health needs, such as epilepsy, challenging behaviour, offending behaviour, dementia, and autistic spectrum disorder (Scottish Executive Health Department, 2002). Indeed, Beange *et al* (1995) suggest that as many as two-thirds of people with learning disabilities require support over and above that provided by primary care alone. Specifically, up to 50% of people with learning disabilities are likely to experience epilepsy (Scottish Executive Health Department, 2002), nearly 17% will display challenging behaviour (Qureshi and Alborz, 1992), up to 5% will present with offending behaviours (Day, 1997), and 45% of people with Down's syndrome over 55 years of age are likely to develop dementia (Visser, 1997).

Valuing People (DoH, 2001) clearly recognises the additional and complex health needs of people with learning disabilities, and sets out a range of specific targets aimed at reducing health inequalities. Once again the role of primary and secondary health care is emphasised, together with calls for an end to discrimination. The applicability of NSFs for mental health, coronary heart disease, older people and diabetes, and the National Cancer Plan, to people with learning disabilities is also accentuated. 'Health facilitators', drawn primarily from community learning disability teams, are seen as the barrier busters, supporting access to other NHS services, wherever necessary, through the medium of 'health action plans'. Greater partnership working is identified as a fundamental priority, in turn requiring a range of training initiatives (DoH, 2001).

Targeting interprofessional education

Roberts (2002) suggests that interprofessional education (IPE) involving nurses should be targeted at two different levels: those currently undergoing pre-registration training and those already practising. However, his assertions are predicated on current structures for the education of health professionals, and do not necessarily take account of plans currently being considered for generic health workers. For example, Humphris and Macleod-Clark (2002) argue that, in order to achieve modernisation, whole system curriculum and practice development reform is required, as opposed to simply 'adding on' to existing programmes. In response, Hale (2002), while supporting the notion of a common core curriculum across all professional groups, counters that professional identity must be retained, and that the agenda for IPE should be on collaboration and not genericism. So, returning to the arguments of Roberts (2002), who needs to collaborate, over what, and at what level?

It is clear from the Scottish Review that all nurses will potentially make an important contribution to the health of people with learning disabilities (Scottish Executive Health Department, 2002). Therefore, experience of caring for this particular client group must be mandatory across common foundation programmes, although the way in which such experience is constructed may vary:

⌘ One university uses 'problem-based learning' [PBL] as a means for students to develop insights into the needs of people with learning disabilities. Through PBL based on real-life scenarios, developed in conjunction with nurses from the local specialist provider, students are required to research issues arising from commonly presenting health needs. Naturally, these include the nursing interventions required, but also explore the respective responsibilities of primary, secondary and specialist services in ensuring that interventions meet need, the barriers to accessing such services, and how involvement and consent on the part of the client can be achieved.

⌘ Another university, in developing a degree-level pre-registration nursing programme, has reached agreement with the local specialist provider that all students, regardless of the branch they intend to pursue, will be required to undertake a two-week learning disability placement. This will include experience with the community team, community residential service, and an acute inpatient unit for people with challenging behaviour and/or mental health needs.

However, as Roberts (2002) asserts, we must also target training at those already practising. Once again, there are a number of examples of how this can be achieved, both through traditional educational means, and through joint work and 'learning on the job':

⌘ Nurses from the local specialist provider have recently made contact with their counterparts in practice nursing. Together they have drawn up a training agenda and are about to embark on a series of reciprocal training sessions. The learning disability nurses want to know more about chronic disease conditions and their management within primary care. The practice nurses are keen to learn about health conditions known to be associated with learning disability, and practical strategies for supporting people with challenging behaviour or mental health difficulties who might attend the surgery.

⌘ A Regional Training Fellow has been appointed, with support from the North and East Yorkshire Workforce Development Confederation, with a remit to identify training needs, share best practice initiatives, raise awareness and promote networking between learning disability nurses and colleagues in acute and primary care. As a result, a cross-sector group of nurses has been established, and a symposium was recently held to share best practice in acute and primary care for people with learning disabilities, attracting a range of GPs, consultants, audiologists together with nurses from private, voluntary and statutory services. A new category of acute/primary care has subsequently been established on the National Network of Learning Disability Nurses' website to allow others to learn from the numerous best practice examples described therein (Kent, 2002).

⌘ Health checks were offered to thirty-five people with learning disabilities through a collaborative project that sought to detect, quantify and treat physical and mental health conditions in the practice population. The health checks took place at the general practice surgery and were conducted by the GP, a consultant psychiatrist in learning disability, and a community learning disability nurse. In addition to identifying physical health needs in 94% of the sample and mental health needs in 25%, the health checks also highlighted the training needs of GPs in relation to communication, consent and compliance (Cassidy *et al*, 2002).

⌘ Learning disability nurses and occupational therapists from the local specialist provider have tried to strengthen links, and develop practice, with colleagues from the mental health division of the trust. A session on the values that underpin practice, based on the principles of normalisation and social role valorisation (Wolfensberger, 1983), has been incorporated into the trust's mental health development programme for support workers. Options for providing clinical supervision to psychiatric nurses caring for people with learning disabilities on inpatient wards are being explored, with a view to enhancing communication skills and understanding of behavioural presentations. Educational sessions have also been delivered to basic grade occupational therapists, with the aim of promoting awareness of issues such as sensory impairment, consent and person-centred care.

⌘ A multi-agency 'forensic interest group' has recently been established by the local specialist provider, with a view to strengthening links and enhancing collaborative working arrangements across the range of services involved in supporting people with learning disabilities at risk of (re)offending. The early work of the group has focused on raising awareness of the respective roles of each of the agencies involved. Following initial training sessions on the recognition of learning disability, the group is now developing plans for 'rolling out' this training to police, probation and prison officers.

Yet one cannot escape the fact that since *Better Services* (DoH, 1971) the prevailing model of care has shifted away from the traditional medical model towards a social construction of disability, with local authorities as the lead service provider (Thompson, 1998). While this does not negate the roles and responsibilities of NHS staff, as can be seen from the above discussion, it does call for a broadening of the concept of IPE. For example, Clarke (1998) cites how, in 1980, the then Secretary of State for Social Services called upon the General Nursing Council and the Council for Education and Training in Social Work to explore the general training needs of staff caring for people with learning disabilities. Nonetheless, policy-makers have been slow to act, with little progress in producing a framework for progress, and an overriding attitude of 'benign neglect' (Clarke, 1998). However, despite a lack of impetus from the top, developments on the ground do give cause for hope:

⌘ Manchester University currently offers a joint social work and learning disability nursing pre-registration programme leading to dual qualification. Students completing the course are then able to opt for a career in either nursing or social care, but remain well placed to influence and support colleagues in either sector in pursuit of enhancing service quality.

⌘ The Royal College of Nursing (RCN) Learning Disability Forum is considering the place and potential of generic care workers in the health and social care of people with a learning disability. As a result of their deliberations, a model for career development, based loosely on the notion of a joint nursing and social work programme, was presented at a fringe event of the RCN Congress 2002. Plans for a further open forum discussion are afoot so as to move from vision to reality.

Examples of the benefits that may be realised through health and social care IPE are clearly evident. For example, it is now recognised that those providing social support for people with learning disabilities are ideally placed to encourage healthier lifestyles and undertake healthcare tasks (DoH, 2001). Matthews *et al* (2002) describe how this may be achieved through use of the 'OK Health Check' – a comprehensive system of health assessment designed specifically for people with learning disabilities, which relies on the reports of the individual's immediate carer (Matthews, 1996). Donnelly and Earnshaw (2002) also report the development of a training programme to raise care workers' awareness of the needs of people with Down's syndrome and Alzheimer's disease. These are but a few examples, which demonstrate how practitioners on the ground are taking forward the agenda on IPE and partnership working.

Conclusion

People with learning disabilities are likely to experience greater health need than their non-disabled counterparts. In addition to the everyday needs experienced by the general population, they are also prone to a range of conditions arising both directly and indirectly from their learning disability, which may be multiple and complex. Following closure of the long-stay hospitals, the vast majority of people with learning disabilities now live in the community and have the same rights of access to mainstream primary care, community and hospital services as any other citizen. However, despite a succession of policy initiatives, there is still overwhelming evidence that uptake of such services is considerably lower than expected. This, at least in part, is attributed to a lack of knowledge pertaining to learning disability on the part of mainstream NHS staff.

The new learning disability strategy *Valuing People* describes a vision of choice, rights, independence and inclusion for people with learning disabilities. Good health is vital to achieving that vision. In order for people with learning disabilities to achieve good health, a range of services and professionals, including mental health, primary and secondary care, social services, the independent sector, and the criminal justice system, must work in partnership, both in practice and in education. Within the current educational structures, there is a need to target those undertaking pre-registration training and those already practising. The potential shift towards generic workers also holds considerable promise, so that in team-working for the future:

> '... *meeting the needs of people with learning disabilities ... [will genuinely] ... become routine good practice and not a problem to be overcome.*'

(Hutton, 1999a)

References

Barker M, Howells G (1990) The medical needs of adults. In: *Primary Care for People with a Mental Handicap*. Occasional Paper No. 47. RCOG, London

Beange H, McElduff A, Baker W (1995) Medical disorders of adults with mental retardation: population study. *Am J Ment Retard* **99**(6): 595–604

Cassidy G, Martin DM, Martin GHB, Roy A (2002) Health checks for people with learning disabilities: community learning disability teams working with general practitioners and primary health care teams. *J Learn Disabil* **6**(2): 123–36

Chaplin R, Flynn A (2000) Adults with learning disability admitted to psychiatric wards. *Advances in Psychiatric Treatment* **6**: 128–34

Clarke SJG (1998) The community as an arena for shared learning and practice. In: Thompson T, Mathias P (Eds). *Standards and Learning Disability*. 2nd edn. Baillière Tindall, London

Cooper SA (1997) Epidemiology of psychiatric disorders in elderly compared with younger adults with learning disabilities. *Br J Psychiatry* **170**: 375–80

Cooper SA, Bailey NM (2001) Psychiatric disorders amongst adults with learning disabilities: prevalence and relationship to ability level. *Irish Journal of Psychological Medicine* **18**: 45–53

Day K (1997) Sex offenders with learning disabilities. In: Read SG (Ed). *Psychiatry in Learning Disability*. WB Saunders, London

Department of Health (1971) *Better Services for the Mentally Handicapped*. DoH, London

Department of Health (1995) *Learning Disability: Meeting Needs through Targeting Skills. A guide to learning disability nursing for health and social care commissioners, GP fundholders, NHS trusts and the independent sector*. DoH, London

Department of Health (1999) *Facing the Facts: Services for People with Learning Disabilities: A policy impact study of social care and health services.* DoH, London.

Department of Health (2001) *Valuing People: A new strategy for learning disability for the 21st century.* DoH, London.

Donnelly V, Earnshaw K (2002) Training for success. *Learning Disability Practice: The Journal for Professionals Working with People with Learning Disabilities* **5** (1): 14–16

Doody G (2001) Mental health services for people with learning disabilities: people with co-morbidity can fall between two stools. *BMJ* **322**: 301

Hale C (2002) *Questioning the Conventional Wisdom.* Leeds University, Leeds

Hardy S, Bouras N (2002) The presentation and assessment of mental health problems in people with learning disabilities. *Learning Disability Practice: The Journal for Professionals Working with People With Learning Disabilities* **5**(3): 33–9

Howells G (1986) Are the medical needs of mentally handicapped adults being met? *J R Coll Gen Pract* **36**: 449–53

Humphris D, Macleod-Clark J (2002) *Shaping a Vision for a 'New Generation' Workforce.* Faculty of Medicine, Health & Biological Sciences, Southampton University, Southampton

Hunt C, Wakefield S, Hunt G (2001) Community nurse learning disabilities: a case study of the use of an evidence-based screening tool to identify and meet the health needs of people with learning disabilities. *J Learn Disabil* **5**(1): 9–18

Hutton J (1999a) Foreword. In: NHS Executive. *Once a Day one or more people with learning disabilities are likely to be in contact with your primary healthcare team. How can you help them?* DoH, London

Hutton J (1999b) *Learning Disability Strategy.* HSC MIS (99)56

Hutton J (2000) Minister outlines plans for learning disability strategy. In: DoH Press release 000/0597

Kay B, Rose S, Turnbull J (1995) *Continuing the Commitment: The report of the learning disability nursing project.* DoH, London

Kent A (2002) Sharing best practice: nurses in A2A see eye 2 eye on championing access to acute care. *Link Up: The Newsletter for all RCN Nurses Working in Learning Disabilities* **Summer** 4–5

Matthews DR (1996) *The OK Health Check.* Fairfield Publications, Preston

Matthews D, Fidler D, Thompson L (2002) A cause for concern. *Learning Disability Practice: The Journal for Professionals Working with People with Learning Disabilities* **5**(1): 10–12

Meehan S, Moore G, Barr O (1995) Specialist services for people with learning disabilities *Nurs Times* **91**(13): 33–5

Moss SC, Prosser H, Costello H, Simpson N, Patel P (1998) Reliability and validity of the PAS-ADD checklist for detecting psychiatric disorders in adults with intellectual disability. *J Intellect Disabil Res* **42**: 173–83

NHS Executive (1998) *Signposts for Success in Commissioning and Providing Health Services for People with Learning Disabilities.* DoH, London

NHS Executive (1999) *Once a Day one or more people with learning disabilities are likely to be in contact with your primary healthcare team: how can you help them?* DoH, London

Qureshi H, Alborz A (1992) Epidemiology of challenging behaviour. *Mental Handicap Research* 5(2): 130–45

Roberts S (2002) Challenging times. *Learning Disability Practice: The Journal for Professionals Working with People With Learning Disabilities* **5**(4): 6

Royal College of Psychiatrists (1996) *Meeting the Mental Health Needs of People with Learning Disability. Council Report CR56.* RCP, London

Scottish Executive Health Department (2002) *The National Review of the Contribution of Nurses to the Care and Support of People with Learning Disabilities: The Complex Needs Subgroup Report.* Scottish Executive, Edinburgh

Social Services Inspectorate (1998) *Moving into the Mainstream: An inspection of services for adults with learning disabilities: a summary report for front-line staff and their managers.* DoH, London

Thompson C (1998) The National Health Service. In: Thompson T, Mathias P (Eds). *Standards and Learning Disability.* 2nd edn. Baillière Tindall, London

Turner S, Moss S (1996). The health needs of adults with learning disabilities and the *Health of the Nation* strategy. *J Intellect Disabil Res* **40**(5): 438–45

Visser N (1997) Ageing and cognitive decline in people with Down's Syndrome. *British Journal of Developmental Disability* **43**: 79–84

Wolfensberger W (1983) Social role valorisation: a proposed new term for the principle of normalisation. *Ment Retard* **21**(6): 234–97

Acknowledgements

My thanks are due to Colin Beacock, Paul Anderton, Dave Matthews, and Dianne Smith for their support in writing this chapter, and for the information provided regarding developments in their respective organisations.

11

Primary care: delivering the modernisation agenda

Kate Cernik and Caroline Carlisle

Primary care teams, comprising a range of healthcare professionals, have worked closely together to deliver care for many years. Recently the boundaries between the scope of practice of these professionals have become more fluid, for example, practice nurses are managing chronic illnesses such as asthma and hypertension. In part, the broadening of responsibilities stemmed from a change in contract in the 1990s for GPs (Department of Health [DoH] and Welsh Office, 1989; Pedersen and Leese, 1997). This required GPs to take on the management of chronic diseases, and financial remuneration was linked to the achievement of target figures of patients attending these clinics. The employment of greater numbers of practice nurses resulted from GPs needing support to achieve targets. Nurses found that taking on new responsibilities enhanced their job satisfaction and often led to further initiatives in patient care management in areas such as the management of the menopause, hormone replacement therapy and travel health.

These changing responsibilities meant that primary healthcare teams had to negotiate their roles and gain a fuller understanding of each other's skills and responsibilities (West and Slater, 1996). Studies have demonstrated that effective multidisciplinary working can lead to improved patient outcomes (Applegate *et al*, 1990; Landefield *et al*, 1995; Brita-Rossi *et al*, 1996). The nature of primary care has fostered a number of innovative approaches to interprofessional education (IPE) in order that more effective multidisciplinary working can be achieved. Indeed, it has been noted that the Royal College of General Practitioners has developed leadership in promoting IPE within the medical profession (Barr, 2001). One reason for this could be the inherent pragmatism in general practice and the need to provide seamless holistic care in the community.

This chapter explores the developments in primary care that have necessitated a more strategic approach to interprofessional learning. Real-life examples from primary care will illustrate a variety of ways that IPE is being introduced, including practice-based learning and multiprofessional implementation of the National Service Framework (NSF) for Mental Health (DoH, 1999) in one NHS primary care trust (PCT).

Developments in primary care

The modernisation of primary care is being driven by the *NHS Plan* (DoH, 2000) in England and Wales, and by *Our National Health* (Scottish Executive, 2001) in Scotland. In primary care, the Plan emphasises the need to improve access to services, and to ensure that the right person delivers the right care in the right place at the right time. A tranche of initiatives have been introduced to achieve this, including NSH Direct (NHS 24 in Scotland), walk-in centres and the National Primary Care Collaborative. These initiatives have been concerned, in the main, with meeting access targets. The NHS Plan also promotes the need to develop interprofessional approaches to education and continuing professional development. More generally, it has been observed that as healthcare systems change, the redesign of healthcare curricula must enhance multiprofessional and community-centred care (Talen *et al,* 1994).

In England, PCTs are responsible for improving the quality of primary care. These new organisations offer the opportunity for developing a comprehensive and strategic approach towards developing education and training in primary care. Primary health-care teams comprise a range of health professionals, including GPs, practice nurses, district nurses, health visitors, community psychiatric nurses, midwives, allied health professionals and counsellors, all of whom are supported by practice managers, administration and reception staff. These teams vary in size according to the registered number of patients. The smallest 'single-handed' GP practices have around 2000 patients, while the larger practices may have up to 25,000 patients.

The scope of primary care has changed rapidly over the past decade. The expanding workload has led to a redistribution of roles and responsibilities within the primary healthcare team. Primary care can be categorised into four main areas: health maintenance; acute illness management; chronic illness management; and the management of increasingly complex presentations. The growth areas in primary care have been in three of these categories: health maintenance, chronic illness management and the management of complex health problems.

The management of chronic illness is influenced by the NSFs, which aim to standardise the quality of care that patients should receive. In order to meet the targets set by the Government in relation to the NSFs, more clinician time is spent on their achievement. This has led to a reduction in available appointments for treating minor illness in GP practices. The Government has responded to such concerns with the creation of 'walk-in' centres, NHS Direct and NHS 24. GP practices have implemented a variety of strategies, including employment of nurse practitioners, nurse triage and telephone consultations, to increase accessibility for patients requiring immediate treatment. All this is occurring at a time when GPs are planning to retire earlier (Kmietowicz, 2001) and fewer GPs are being recruited and trained (Lambert *et al,* 2002).

The blurring of traditional role boundaries has provided one solution to these challenges, and has enabled the nurse's role in primary care to extend and develop in creative ways for the benefit of patients. Nurses are increasingly taking on more of the primary care workload. In terms of the management of acute care, nurse-led telephone triage has enabled practices to enhance access to care (Oldham, 2002). Nurses are now working in extended roles managing episodes of care that include the prescribing of medication in the management of acute care, through extended prescribing and, in the management of chronic illness, supplementary prescribing. Complex problems frequently present in primary care and are dealt with mainly by GPs. However, nurses often work across health communities delivering specialist care in the management of conditions such as rheumatoid arthritis and heart failure. These nurses frequently work closely with colleagues in secondary care and may receive referrals from all members of the primary care team. Thus the workload balance is shifting, with nurses taking on new tasks and roles. These approaches give GPs more time to manage complex conditions and develop their own specialist skills, reducing the need for referral to secondary care (Gerada *et al,* 2002).

In addition, the opportunities presented by new information technology continue to influence teamwork in primary care. Historically, professional groups within primary care have developed their own record-keeping systems — both paper and electronic. Delivering the new NHS agenda requires all primary care clinicians to collaborate on record-keeping. Learning together to maximise the potential of electronic records is a high priority for primary care organisations, as this will promote high-quality transparent practice from all clinicians involved in a patient's care, and reduce fragmentation.

Learning in primary care

Integrated and shared care is a particular goal across both acute and primary care. In primary care there are some very specific reasons why shared care should be a priority. Evidence suggests that interprofessional learning can enhance collaborative working and the development of a more integrated care pathway to a greater extent than uni-professional approaches to continuing development (Barr, 2001). Involvement in learning activities where all participants are required to work together to solve clinical problems, support each other in reflecting on individual professional decisions, and debate who might be the most appropriate professional in the team to manage key problems or issues will encourage teamwork. The 'added value' of IPE can also be an increased awareness of each other's role, with the potential of building respect for the contribution of each team member (NHS Executive South West, 1999). There are potential benefits of IPE to both the patient and healthcare professional:

- each professional is enabled to make full use of his or her skills
- risk management can be recognised as a team responsibility

- role overlap is minimised, thereby saving time for patients and ensuring more effective use of resources
- individual job satisfaction is improved by enabling health professionals to work safely and effectively
- a climate of trust between professionals can be generated
- working relationships are improved by increased understanding of other professional roles and perspectives
- it helps individuals to acquire new skills
- team-working is promoted
- 'crossover' of skills, knowledge and attitudes is encouraged.

Unfortunately, there are also a number of barriers to successful IPE. Power varies between different professional groups. Different employers, role conflict and hierarchical management can lead to real difficulties in obtaining training. For example, while most GPs are good employers committed to staff training, a minority do not release their staff or fund additional learning, which means that these nurses often finance essential training themselves and undertake it in their own time. There are huge variations in the financial support allocated to different professional groups. For example, GPs have more training income per head than nurses; and within nursing there are also huge differentials between different health authorities' commitment to funding and between different groups of nurses.

Professional groups have different strengths and weaknesses, which can make traditional courses and approaches to learning inappropriate. GPs are graduates with a relatively consistent knowledge base, whereas nurses are much more heterogeneous in terms of educational background and experience, and hence often lack confidence in a multiprofessional arena. Long-held beliefs about the characteristics of different professional groups can affect multiprofessional learning between trust- and practice-employed staff, who often have little appreciation of the constraints of the organisations that employ them. While most professions require evidence of continuing professional development to maintain registration, the amount and level of educational activity required varies considerably. Professional groups experience different ways of learning; from apprenticeships to academic study, this has considerable implications for educators.

Four case studies that describe a variety of practical real-life examples of implementing IPE in primary care will now be presented. The advantages of the various approaches and some of the challenges that confronted the clinicians involved in implementing the learning programmes are highlighted.

Case study 1: Improving consultation skills through interprofessional workshops

Background

Effective communication provides the foundation for effective consulting. This is particularly important in primary care where relationships often need to be developed quickly in order to provide an effective therapeutic environment for consultations (Pendleton *et al*, 1984). More nurses are now making use of the consultation model in their own practice because of the developing scope of practice in general practice, walk-in centres, and other nurse-led initiatives.

Learning activity

The Liverpool Postgraduate General Practice Office is responsible for delivering the vocational training scheme for GPs. It runs a highly successful in-house course in communication skills training, originally developed for GPs. The course uses an experiential and reflective model involving simulated patients and video recording of consultations. Over the last 10 years the course has implemented an IPE model and has been attended by nurses, dentists, occupational therapists, physiotherapists, health visitors, midwives, radiographers, managers, receptionists and psychologists, as well as GPs and hospital doctors. Professionals conduct an interaction, normally 10 minutes, based on their everyday activity. A structured debriefing then takes place in a small multiprofessional group of around three other participants with two facilitators and a process observer. The simulated patient contributes to the learning process both in and out of role. Aspects of communication and teaching are explored during this process. Each participant conducts a consultation. The ethical and practical implications of using video-technique in real-life clinical practice are also covered.

What worked well

⌘ The use of multiprofessional groups and facilitators enables participants to recognise the universal nature of communication and consultation skills.

⌘ The process enables participants to observe and debate a variety of professional approaches within differing clinical scenarios.

⌘ The programme provides a unique opportunity to observe other professionals in what is normally an unobserved activity.

⌘ The use of learner-centred approaches ensures that in a multiprofessional group every participant develops an awareness of his or her strengths and has opportunities to explore ways of doing things differently.

⌘ The enthusiasm and commitment of a team of multiprofessional facilitators has generated a dynamic programme that has responded flexibly to the changing needs of a diverse range of professionals.

What we learned

⌘ Publicity material should avoid being professional biased.
⌘ Learning resources, such as case studies, should be appropriate to all professional groups.
⌘ Professional language and jargon should be avoided.
⌘ Because of differing funding streams, mechanisms need to be developed to enable non-doctors to access the course.
⌘ Publicity networks are less well developed for allied health professions and nurses – this issue still needs addressing.
⌘ Residential courses may present difficulties for parents.
⌘ Professional experiences and expectations need to be accounted for in developing the programmes.

Case study 2: An approach to practice-based learning

Background

Appleton primary care is a first-wave personal medical services (PMS) pilot in a greenfield site, which provides primary care services to more than 2000 patients. The multiprofessional team includes a GP, nurse clinician and primary care nurse. The team is employed by Warrington primary care trust and is self-managing. It contracts for clinical services with the strategic health authority. It makes use of computerised electronic records. The team strives to innovate in the delivery of services; for example, it has developed patient-held records (Khong *et al,* 2000).

In addition, each team member has access to a desktop computer. A healthcare navigation site has been developed by the team, which provides team members with the opportunity to search for healthcare information either when the patient is present or to meet their own learning needs.

Learning activity

As part of the Practice and Professional Development Plan, weekly education meetings are held for clinical staff. The meetings provide an opportunity for the team to discuss a range of clinical issues, including problem cases, random cases (a presentation of a consultation undertaken by a team member that day), significant events or significant 'hot' topics. Ground rules have been established; these include appropriate confidentiality, openness and honesty, and the use of non-judgmental language.

Clinicians normally take turns to present a topic, and other team members then discuss issues arising from it. The outcome varies according to the topic, but may result in:

- revised management planning for patients
- new learning needs for team members
- generation of team learning tasks
- sharing of clinical information
- literature review.

A summary of each meeting is e-mailed to each team member. This can be included in the professional's portfolio, which each team member maintains as a record of his or her learning activities. This approach facilitates the auditing of learning activities, to ensure that practice goals are achieved.

What worked well

⌘ A 'whole team' approach encourages consistent approaches to clinical management of individual patient and of clinical problems.

⌘ Discussion of clinical issues with the whole team fosters trust, which is a key factor in the development of a multiprofessional team.

⌘ The session offers an opportunity for clinicians to share their skills and knowledge, thereby helping individuals to acknowledge the boundaries of their scope of practice.

⌘ Clinicians have the opportunity to reflect on their own practice, reinforcing their strengths and enabling them to identify and address any weaknesses.

⌘ Sharing knowledge acquired at meetings and training courses is a cost-effective use of clinicians' time.

⌘ The process identifies skill gaps in the team as a whole.

⌘ The meetings contribute to the management of risk in the organisation as a whole.

What we learned

⌘ The meetings require dedicated time outside consultation sessions and lunch hours.

⌘ Meetings need to be developed to enable part-time staff to attend.

⌘ Learning is more effective if pressing patient problems or clinicians' anxieties are dealt with first.

⌘ Learning is more effective when ground rules are set.

⌘ Recording of meeting content reinforces learning and ensures that clinicians who have been unable to attend have an opportunity to learn and 'catch-up' if necessary.

Case study 3: Protected primary care education in Liverpool (PROPEL)

Background

A new initiative in Liverpool aimed at supporting clinical excellence through education and professional development was launched in September 2001. The Protected Primary Care Education in Liverpool (PROPEL) Scheme was developed to support learning in practice teams. This was to be achieved by providing protected time for the exchange of ideas and sharing of best practice. The first scheme of this type was developed in Doncaster, and today many similar schemes are being set up across the UK.

The scheme provides the opportunity to discuss local health needs as a series of half-day afternoon sessions held each month in different parts of the city. Some GP surgeries close for the half-day to allow the full staff team to learn together and plan service improvements.

Topics are selected from suggestions put forward by primary healthcare team members, clinical governance leads and other members of PCTs who support practice development. Patient-centred care is the focus of discussion at many events, with patient involvement included in programmes as appropriate. Topics covered have included:

• the NSF for Older People
• coronary heart disease
• women's health
• protecting the child
• violence and aggression in the workplace.

Personnel from social and voluntary services have approached PROPEL to attend topic-specific events; as a result, an 'all-inclusive' approach to attendance has developed. This has led to a wide range of healthcare professionals and others accessing continued professional development opportunities through PROPEL. It is anticipated that the others will wish to attend future events with the expansion of the integrated health and social care agenda. PROPEL is keen to promote the shared care approach to learning by involving professionals from both primary and secondary care in contributing to this education programme. Bringing together the many different groups will help all staff to share best practice and learn about new innovations in the NHS.

PROPEL is supported by a GP advisor, nurse education advisor, practice staff education advisor and an administrator. The day-to-day management of the scheme is the responsibility of a coordinator. A 'pool' of multiprofessional facilitators has been trained to assist in delivery of the events.

Learning activity

The delivery style varies from workshops, lectures, discussion groups to the use of drama groups in role-play. A three-hour programme may contain a mix of learning styles to support large audience and small group participation. At the events, delegates are presented with a pack containing a source of PGEA approval is obtained and all delegates receive a certificate of attendance.Delegates are encouraged to develop a learning portfolio and copies of learning evaluations are made available. The protected learning time scheme is now moving towards promoting and encouraging practices to organise their own in-practice event. Assistance in the planning and design of the programme, facilitation and funding is available.

What worked well

⌘ Multi- and uni-professional groups working and learning together.
⌘ Developing a multiprofessional team of facilitators models multiprofessional ways of working.
⌘ Problem-based learning, using clinical case studies, has proved a popular method for learning and sharing best practice across the professions.
⌘ The involvement of other non-NHS organisations in planning and delivery has brought a wider perspective to the topics.
⌘ Involving both sectors in the delivery of events has strengthened communication between primary and secondary care.

What we learned

- ⌘ Bringing together a range of disciplines from across the primary care field contributes to sharing 'best practice' and learning about new innovations. The importance of promoting a team-working approach.
- ⌘ How to acknowledge different learning styles and encompass these in the delivery and design of the events. This is particularly important when both clinical and support and administrative staff attend events.
- ⌘ The importance of expert facilitators.
- ⌘ The contribution from local experts, from both primary and secondary care, is vital to the success of the events.
- ⌘ Some practices find it easier to attend than others; non-attendance may be due to time pressure or a perception that the topics are not relevant.
- ⌘ Practice-based learning should be targeted at those practices that have attendance problems.

Case study 4: Integrated care pathways for mental health

Background

Integrated care pathways (ICPs) enable the mapping of the patient's journey with the delivery of services, underpinned by guidance from best evidence and local flexibility. It is a way of measuring concordance and developing new ways of working.

Trafford North and South Primary Care Trusts in partnership with Trafford Health Care Trust and the local Mental Health Partnership collaborated on this programme. This involved setting up a project team represented by stakeholders in the programme, literature searching and compiling, and understanding the steps taken both by patient and health professionals in managing mental health conditions.

Learning activity

The first step was to explain the concept of ICPs and the nature of the programme. Feedback from these stakeholder sessions enabled the production of a draft ICP in depression, a common and familiar condition in general practice.

The next step was to identify general practices that wished to pilot the draft ICP and a training needs assessment (TNA). A matrix of larger/smaller and inner urban/suburban practices were selected. The assessment sought to identify barriers to delivering an ICP and any weakness in the pathway. The outcomes of the TNA were used to design the approach to disseminating the ICP and accompanying support to general practice and primary care mental health teams. The result is a staged implementation process.

Initially a stakeholder event was held to launch the ICPs in mental health. The production of an information pack and learning resource in the form of a CD-ROM was then developed collaboratively with a pharmaceutical company. This pack includes:

- an introduction to ICPs
- DoH strategy
- education
- documents
- patient information.

Other parts of the package provide clinicians with educational tools such as:

- NSF standards
- Trafford ICP
- educational materials on the management of depression and psychoses
- local referral networks
- local care pathways.

All clinicians have access to the same learning resources and will be encouraged to make use of them as part of an IPE approach. Such an approach also provides an opportunity for mental health workers to be supported in their attempts to implement change. The same resources can be used for specialised groups who deliver the ICP, such as health visitors and GPs.

What worked well

- ⌘ Having a single point of contact for the development and design of the ICP.
- ⌘ Having educational support for the project coordinator. This ensures a structured educational approach to implementation of the ICP, including taking appropriate objectives, such as attitudinal change, into account.
- ⌘ Linking the multimedia CD-ROM with local personal development programmes, including educational accreditation.
- ⌘ Targeting small group workshops for specialised areas of the ICPs.
- ⌘ Personal delivery and input of the project coordinator to each practice.

What we learned

- ⌘ An educational approach is time-consuming, both in planning and execution.

⌘ There is much synergy in taking an educational approach to ICP development and its implementation.

⌘ Key stakeholders and opinion leaders need to be engaged early for project credibility and spread.

⌘ Leadership is required to ensure sustainability and focus.

⌘ Working with industry partners can be rewarding so long as probity arrangements/expectations are in place.

Conclusions

The four case studies outlined above are practical examples of a commitment to IPE in primary care. The importance of teamwork in primary care has long been recognised by successive governments in White Papers and policy documents. (DoH and Welsh Office [WO], 1989, 2000, 2002a). The development of PCTs offer the professions more opportunities to engage in 'joined-up' learning, as managerial and funding barriers are removed. A variety of initiatives are underway, and these should continue to foster strategic approaches to education for all practitioners. For example, the DoH (2000) and the Royal College of General Practitioners (RCGP) (2002) recommend that practitioners have individualised learning plans in place, and that these learning plans respond to the needs of the organisation as well as the needs of individual clinicians (DoH, 2002b; RCGP, 2002). Practice, work-based education provides the opportunity for closer teamwork and local responsiveness to health issues. E-learning, team learning and shared approaches to service delivery have enabled the Appleton team to improve patient care. New opportunities to continue this work will be presented by the expanded role of nurses and pharmacists in particular; for example, a shared approach to the education required for medicines management appears to make good sense as the number of prescribers is likely to grow as extended and supplementary prescribing expands (DoH, 2002c).

The responsibility of PCTs to deliver sound clinical governance has fostered a number of collaborative education initiatives such as those described above. Such initiatives explicitly acknowledge that education has a strategic role in delivering both clinical and organisational imperatives. The added value of an interprofessional approach to these initiatives has resulted in a greater understanding of the role and scope of practice of respective members of the primary healthcare team. Additionally, there is exciting potential for future research which can demonstrate the value of these educational activities using outcome measures such as risk reduction, access, client/patient satisfaction and prescribing behaviour.

References

Applegate SB, Miller ST, Graney MJ, Elam JT, Burns R, Akins DE (1990) A randomised controlled trial of a geriatric assessment unit in a community rehabilitation hospital. *N Engl J Med* **322**: 1572–8

Barr H (2001) *Interprofessional Education: Today, yesterday and tomorrow*. UK Centre for the Advancement of Interprofessional Education (CAIPE), London

Brita-Rossi P, Adduci D, Kaufman J, Lipson SJ, Totte C, Wasserman K (1996) Improving the process of care: the cost, quality, value of interdisciplinary collaboration. *J Nurs Care Qual* **10**(2): 10–16

Department of Health and Welsh Office (1989) *General Practice in the NHS: A new contract*. DHSS, London

Department of Health (1999) *A National Service Framework for Mental Health*. The Stationery Office, London

Department of Health (2000) *The NHS Plan. A plan for investment. A plan for reform*. The Stationery Office, London

Department of Health (2002a) Achieving and sustaining improved access to primary care. www.doh.gov.uk/pricare/improvedacccess.htm (accessed 21 February 2003)

Department of Health (2002b) *Improved Working Lives*. The Stationery Office, London

Department of Health (2002c) *Extending Independent Nurse Prescribing within the NHS in England – A guide for implementation*. The Stationery Office, London

Gerada C, Wright N, Keen J (2002) The general practitioner with a special interest: new opportunities or the end of the generalist practitioner? *Br J Gen Pract* **52**: 796–8

Kmietowicz Z (2001) Quarter of GPs want to quit BMA survey shows. *BMJ* **323**: 887

Lambert TW, Evans J,Goldacre MJ (2002) Recruitment of UK-trained doctors into general practice: findings from national cohort studies. *Br J Gen Pract* **52**: 364–7, 369–72

Landefield CS, Palmer RM, Kresevic DM, Fortinsky RH, Kowal J (1995) A randomised trial of care in a hospital medical unit especially designed to improve the functional outcomes of acutely ill older patients. *N Engl J Med* **332**: 1338–44

NHS Executive South West (1999) *Achieving Health and Social Care Improvements through Interprofessional Education*. Institute of Health and Community Studies, Bournemouth University

Oldham J (2002) Telephone use in primary care (Letter). *BMJ* **325**: 547

Pedersen LL, Leese B (1997) What will a primary care led NHS mean for GP workload? The problem of the lack of an evidence base. *BMJ* **314**: 1337–41

Pendleton D, Schofield T, Tate P, Havelock P (1984) *The Consultation: An approach to learning and teaching*. Oxford University Press, Oxford

Royal College of General Practitioners and General Practitioners Committee (2002) *Good Medical Practice for General Practitioners*. RCGP/GPC, London

Scottish Executive (2001) *Our National Health. A plan for action. A plan for change*. The Scottish Office, Edinburgh

Talen MR, Graham MC, Walbroehl G (1994) Introducing multiprofessional team practice and community-based health care services into the curriculum: a challenge for health care educators. *Family Systems Medicine* **12**(4): 353–60

West MA, Slater J (1996) *Team-working in Primary Health Care: A review of its effectiveness.* Health Education Authority, London

12

Interprofessional learning: context, meaning and technology

Di Marks-Maran and Gill Young

Much has been written about different approaches to learning. However, the literature relating to the development and delivery of interprofessional and electronic learning contains little on how alternative approaches to learning might influence the design, approach to and delivery of the curriculum. This chapter posits 'constructivism' as a theory about learning and its relationship to practice – the key place where expertise is developed, with skilled practitioners acting as facilitators. Learning and teaching are therefore concerned with the development of professional knowledge, understanding and competence. The chapter will begin with a discussion of constructivism as a theory about learning that can guide the development and delivery of interprofessional and online learning in health care.

In 1997 the Faculty of Health and Human Sciences at Thames Valley University (TVU) made a strategic decision to revisit its approaches to learning and teaching, and to enable academic staff to explore a range of theories about learning and their impact on the planning and delivery of educational programmes. Many of the academic staff, it emerged, had been using a range of methods to deliver their programmes, and modules, that reflected constructivism. Until this point, however, the Faculty had no strategic statement about its corporate approach to learning and teaching. In developing distance and e-learning, we wanted to ensure that these initiatives were driven by an understanding of learning processes, rather than being dictated by the technology available to us.

Two case studies are presented to support and illustrate the discussion. The first is a multiprofessional, social constructivist, learning project. The second began as a uniprofessional web-based project, but following evaluation offers the potential for multiprofessional web-based learning.

Background

The Faculty of Health and Human Sciences at Thames Valley University is one of the largest providers of nursing and midwifery education in the UK. Some 290 academic staff and 90 administrators support approximately 2500 pre-registration nursing and midwifery students and 2750 post-registration students. We work with two NHS Workforce Development Confederations and more than 20 NHS primary and acute care trusts from central London down the Thames Valley to Newbury in Berkshire. Students undertake practice (workplace) experience in some 1200 placements (for example, wards, health centres and clinics) where they are taught, supervised and assessed by thousands of healthcare staff.

The Faculty has been collaborating with three other higher education institutions (Imperial College of Science, Technology and Medicine; Buckinghamshire Chiltern University College; Brunel University) over the last three years to establish clinical, interprofessional education (IPE) for some undergraduate students, in the form of an initiative called the Joint Undergraduate Multiprofessional Project (JUMP). Through this experience, we have gained an understanding of the barriers to IPE and developed strategies or solutions to address these.

The Faculty is engaged with the West London Workforce Development Confederation to build on this work, establishing interprofessional learning for undergraduate and newly qualified healthcare students, and teachers, at all West London trusts and higher education institutions.

Another factor influencing the Faculty's continuing development in both interprofessional learning and e-learning is the Learning Communities Development (LCD) commenced in 2001/02. This initiative builds on, consolidates and coordinates previous innovations aimed at improving the experience of pre- and post-registration nursing and midwifery students, such as practice-based education, problem-based learning and the JUMP project. The principles underpinning the 'learning communities' development are still emerging. This development brings together theories and thinking from several sources. Work on learning organisations (Senge, 1990; Senge *et al*, 1994, 1999; Tosey, 1999; Clarke 2001; Senge, 2002) has been the major influence, a learning organisation being:

> '...an organisation with an ingrained philosophy for anticipating, reacting and responding to change, complexity and uncertainty'
>
> (Malhotra, 1996: 2)

Such organisations are characterised by an openness to new ideas and creativity, an empowered workforce, collaborative approaches, and working in appropriately sized teams to enable effective communication (Mohr and Dichter, 2001). In a learning community, authority is shared within an open culture where staff are facilitated and empowered to take local responsibility for decision-making (Prestine, 1993). Other bodies of work have also impacted on this development, including 'situated learning' (Lave and Wenger, 1991), 'communities of practice' (Wenger, 1998) and 'social constructivism' (Vygotsky, 1978). These form the theoretical frameworks for learning and teaching in the Faculty's nursing and midwifery programmes.

The Faculty of Health and Human Sciences at Thames Valley University, and its related NHS trusts, are using the principles of 'learning organisation theory and practice' to challenge traditional working relationships. This involves moving from the position of a higher education institution working in partnership primarily with its NHS trusts (employers), to a position in which all activity in a geographical location related to the quality of the student experience embraces all the stakeholder organisations and agencies. These bodies form an interdependent learning community, which can learn and adapt its systems to produce practitioners 'fit for purpose and practice' (United Kingdom Central Council for Nursing, Midwifery and Health Visiting [UKCC], 1999).

Context

Constructivism is based on the premise that people construct an existent universe that cannot be known apart from their knowing activity. In other words, you cannot separate 'what' is learned from 'how' it is learned and used (Brown *et al*, 1998). This is in complete contrast to the traditional view of learning, which holds that there is an independently existing universe 'out there' with knowledge that describes, reflects and corresponds to that world. This traditional view assumes:

> '... *a separation between knowing and doing, treating knowledge as an integral, self-sufficient substance, theoretically independent of the situations in which it is learned and used.'*
>
> (Brown *et al*, 1998: 1)

In contructivism the emphasis is on what is happening to the student rather than what the teacher is doing, and through an interaction with objects, events and people the student gains an understanding (meaning) of these. Learning is the result of mental construction, and students learn by fitting new information together with what they already know. The context, the beliefs and the attitudes of the student effect learning, and the student is encouraged to invent his or her own solutions and try out ideas and hypotheses.

Thus, constructivism is interested in the ways that students create meaning from their learning experiences. Learning is not just receiving, storing and retrieving information: it is an internal process of interpretation leading to meaning for that individual. Nor is learning simply the transferring of knowledge from the external world into the memory of the student. Instead, learners create interpretations of the world, and of new knowledge, based on their previous experiences and their interactions with the world.

This approach does not deny the existence of an objective, measurable reality, but it does question the existence of objective knowledge. Constructivists would argue that there are multiple ways to structure the world, and multiple interpretations or meanings for any event or concept. Learning must therefore be durable, transferable and self-regulated. The whole concept of 'lifelong learning' is based on a constructivist perspective to learning, and the student needs to develop deep internal mental processes to facilitate this experience.

Within constructivism there are two main schools of thought – 'social' and 'cognitive' constructivism – although both reflect the same basic assumptions about learning. Cognitive constructivism owes its beginnings to Piaget (1972) who believed that learning is a complex process of assimilation, accommodation and equilibrium. However, here we will concentrate on social constructivism, derived from the work of Vygotsky (1978) and emphasising the influence of cultural and social contexts in learning. This supports a 'discovery model' of learning, which places the teacher in the role of one who creates learning experiences and opportunities that enable students' mental abilities to develop, naturally, through various paths of discovery.

Vygotsky (1978) further suggests that there are three principal assumptions within social constructivism:

⌘ *Making meaning* — the community in which the student lives and works plays a central role, and the people around the student greatly affect the way an individual student sees the world.

⌘ *Tools for cognitive development* — the type and quality of the tools for cognitive development determine the pattern and rate of development in the student. These include important people in the student's working or social life, culture and language.

⌘ *The zone of proximal development* — problem-solving skills related to tasks can be placed into three categories: those performed independently by the student; those that cannot be performed even with help; and those that fall between these two extremes (problem-solving tasks that can be performed with help).

The above model correlates with Renshaw's (1995) socio-cultural model of learning, where it is proposed that:

* learning is social
* teaching is a joint activity
* learning is assisted performance
* teaching is guided conversation
* learning is interactive and co-constructive
* learning is self-regulation among the group
* teaching is helping joint constructions to form
* learning is evaluating shared values
* teaching is enacting community values.

Social constructivism posits that learning is a social and collaborative activity that cannot be 'taught', and it is up to the student to construct his or her own understandings. The teacher's 'job':

> *'... is to "broker" a learning environment that supports the learning activities appropriate to achieving the desired learning outcomes.'*
> (Biggs, 1999)

Social constructivism requires that mechanisms be built into the curriculum so that the assessment and delivery methods are aligned with each other (Biggs, 1999), fostering collaboration between learners. This ultimately creates an environment in which:

> *'... the learner finds it difficult to escape without learning.'*
> (Biggs, 1999)

Two separate case studies are discussed below. These illustrate the use of two approaches to teaching and learning which operationalise Renshaw's (1995) socio-cultural model, and have their philosophical roots in constructivism.

⌘ The first demonstrates how the use of problem-based learning was a key component in the success of an interprofessional learning initiative.

⌘ The second uses the Interpretation Construction (ICON) design (Black and McClintock, 1995) for the development and delivery of an adult nursing intensive care course supported by distance learning.

Case study 1: Joint Undergraduate Multiprofessional Project [JUMP]

JUMP was funded by the NHS Executive (NHSE) from 1999-2001, with the aim of extending medical students' understanding of other healthcare professions through the development of multiprofessional education projects. It centred on medical students at Imperial College School of Medicine when they were on clinical attachments at two West London hospitals. The programmes, conducted during clinical placements, included senior staff on site at the hospitals with staff and students from other professions and universities. Although this initiative has been called 'multiprofessional', most of the activity has been interprofessional, in that students of one profession learn from staff and students of other professions on an interactive, small group basis.

A typical programme consisted of a group of six to eight students who attended three sessions, or participated in activities, over a three-week period. For example, medical and nursing students in one project were required to work in 'medical-nursing student pairs' to take a clinical and social history from a patient, followed by a discussion of their assessment with a specialist nurse involved in the patient's care. In the last session the student pair jointly presented their assessment findings to their peers and the teaching team. For some medical students, this was the first time they realised that nurses collected different history data from patients and the reasons why. In another project, where medical students were developing history-taking skills, they took histories from elderly care patients, and then discussed their assessment findings and conclusions with an occupational therapist, rather than medical staff, as had previously been the case.

A project manager, seeking willing 'guinea pigs', initiated the projects. This was usually a consultant or specialist registrar, who then invited other clinical team members to join the project as co-teachers/facilitators. In the 'diabetes mellitus project', for example, the consultant, the diabetes specialist nurse and the dietitian jointly organised and co-taught the sessions. An external lecturer trained the clinical team as teachers and helped them develop their initial problem-based learning scenarios. Once teams became confident in teaching together, using interactive learning techniques and designing scenarios, little outside assistance or management was required. Some staff had already attended sessions in problem-based learning run by Imperial College, and staff learnt from each other as they became familiar with working as part of a teaching team.

Initially, many of the staff felt unhappy about letting 'their' students be taught by members of another profession, so all attended and took part in teaching the sessions. This was very labour intensive; however, it resulted in them hearing one another's contributions. Most teams were willing, and in fact had assumed they would be repeating the material. As time went on, team members became more confident about teaching together, and took it in turn to attend the sessions. Teams were usually willing and enthusiastic to hear the student evaluations, and modifications were made in the light of this feedback and because of staff changes.

These were very much 'ground up' projects, and the success of JUMP depended on the commitment of key players who, from the outset, acted as internal product champions in each of the hospitals. Momentum and knowledge of JUMP quickly spread, as students enjoyed the experience and found it useful. The biggest difficulty was gaining information about attachment/placement dates for students from four very different universities, and then finding times when the participating students and staff could come together in the same place and at the same time. The organisational management of JUMP depended very much on having a full-time project manager to carry out administration issues such as setting up the teaching teams, identifying and informing the students from various professions, booking rooms, and conducting review meetings with the teaching teams.

A multiprofessional evaluation group researched this initiative. Activity centred on gathering more information on the attitudes, and changes in attitude, of the staff and students taking part. Evaluation research data were collected and analysed using both quantitative and qualitative methods. Six data collection approaches were used, with varying degrees of success. Below we describe two tools developed to evaluate JUMP and its findings.

Attitudes questionnaire

The attitudes questionnaire, based on the results of focus groups held at the outset and refined through factor analysis, was given out to 849 students. Overall, the students' attitude to multiprofessional learning was very positive. Significant differences were found in attitudes between nursing and medical students, and between medical students starting their clinical training following an intercalated science degree and those who had not done an intercalated BSc. Small, but statistically significant differences in response to some of the questions were found in responses before and after students had participated in JUMP teaching. This tool is now being used to research other IPE projects.

Evaluation matrix

An evaluation matrix was developed for any JUMP activity involving several professions, where the possible 'types' of staff were shown at the head of each column and the 'tasks' to be performed in managing the patient under discussion were indicated in the rows. The students were asked to indicate their understanding of which professions were involved in which tasks ('wholly responsible', 'partly responsible', or 'no involvement') at the outset of the activity, and then again at the end. The use of this matrix was, however, reduced after it was discovered that there was as much discrepancy among the staff in their understanding of their colleagues' roles as there was among the students. This finding, though, is interesting in itself, and at least one teaching team is hoping to use the matrix as a tool on which to focus discussion at a regional professional meeting.

From this evaluation, we learnt that the assumption that getting a multiprofessional team to teach together will automatically increase student's understanding of professional roles is false. In one of the JUMP projects where teachers could agree a 'standard', there was evidence that medical students taught by a multiprofessional team did gain a better appreciation of roles of the disciplines involved.

JUMP has provided us with very valuable lessons for the continued development of interprofessional learning and teaching, and the development of robust tools to evaluate the effects of future IPE initiatives. Finally, interviews and observation of the JUMP project revealed that most of the teachers and students involved enjoyed the interprofessional learning experiences — expressing a willingness to take part again.

In 2002, JUMP 2 commenced, funded by the West London Workforce Development Confederation, and aimed at bringing together, where practicable, the clinical training of pre-qualification health professionals. A major goal was to broaden their understanding of care as a process, and to enable them to understand the contribution of other healthcare professionals. As with the original JUMP project, students will be working in small interprofessional groups using enquiry/problem-based learning. Work will also be undertaken to embed interprofessional learning in the curricula.

Case study 2: Developing an online distance learning course in intensive care nursing

In March 1999, the Faculty was awarded an Educational Development Grant to develop and deliver, as a pilot scheme, an online adult intensive care nursing course by supported distance learning. The project was a joint initiative between the Faculty, the English National Board (ENB) and the Open Learning Foundation [OLF]. We chose a highly technical clinical course for this pilot project because many in the healthcare education community have expressed the opinion that online and distance learning is fine for non-clinical/non-technical courses, but not for highly technical clinical programmes. We wanted to test whether the knowledge component of a technically complex clinical specialism could be effectively and efficiently delivered online. Although this was a uniprofessional online development, it has given us a template to use for similar multiprofessional programme design and delivery.

The learning materials were developed and an electronic learning support platform was selected during 2000. The course went 'live' in October 2000 and was delivered in tandem with a separate classroom-based intensive care course. The Faculty's reader in educational development undertook an evaluative research study of the pilot project. The course leader (one of the authors) was also a member of the steering group, which included representatives from the TVU Faculty, the ENB and OLF, two NHS executives, and an external academic from another university. The course was designed as a competency and work-based programme, using a combination of the ICON model (Black and McClintock, 1995) and the situated learning model (Brown *et al*, 1998).

Since the course was built around clinical experience, it was important that students on the pilot programme had access to the online materials and learning support while at work. This involved a partnership agreement with the trusts to purchase and install appropriate hardware and software, on a dedicated PC situated in both of the pilot intensive care unit sites. This enabled the students and their clinical preceptors to access learning materials, email, bulletin boards and online discussion groups. A training programme and induction for clinical preceptors and students was provided.

The ICON model, based on Vygotskian (Vygotsky,1978) or social constructivist learning, was a useful tool to guide the development of learning activities, materials and support for this course. We focused on creating a social collaborative learning environment that was situated in the workplace and promoted learning as a social, interactive process. In recognition that learners make connections with knowledge (or knowledges) in different ways, it was imperative that we built into the course multiple ways of learning and multiple representations of knowledge. Particular emphasis was placed on the social and cultural context in which learning takes place, and how we could enable students to find personal meaning through engaging in practices, discourses and interactions with peers and colleagues. Indeed, the online activities promoted interaction between the learner and objects, events and people to facilitate learning and understanding of adult intensive care nursing.

The electronic learning environment we chose at the time (1999) was the Extended Learning Environment Network (ELEN), which had been developed by a consortium of universities through the Teaching and Learning Technology Programme (TLTP). Thames Valley University was already involved in piloting ELEN as a means of providing online study skills, so it was a natural progression for us to move to using this system to deliver subject-based content and materials. A feature of the learning activities built into the online programme is the use of authentic learning tasks embedded in problem-solving, and relevant to the real-world context of adult intensive care nursing in terms of knowledge and skills. These learning activities encourage sharing, questioning, critiquing, analysing, and the application of new knowledge with reflection on practice.

The evaluative research project of the pilot was undertaken using a realistic evaluation methodology (Pawson and Tilley, 1997). This particular approach was selected because it is appropriate for investigating the introduction of new programmes and delivery methods in 'real-world' situations. Rather than ask 'Does it work or not?', the question becomes 'What is it about the programme that works for whom and in what circumstances?' The purpose of realistic evaluation it is to improve educational programmes or policies. The research involved collection and analysis of data relating to the context, mechanisms and outcomes of the course. Additional questions asked included:

- what impact has the course had on both students and preceptors?
- what impact has this online course had on the clinical environment?
- what was useful in ELEN, and what was not?

Data were gathered through student and preceptor questionnaires, SWOT (strengths, weaknesses, opportunities, threats) analysis, interviews with clinical managers, group interviews with teachers/course designers, learning support and administrative staff, focus group discussion with online and 'taught' students, standard student module evaluations and student assessment results. Analysis of the data was based on grounded theory (Strauss and Corbin, 1990; Boulton and Hammersley, 1996) because much of it was unstructured and in the affective domain. Participants' answers to interview questions were analysed for stable characteristics and recurrent patterns. The key findings of the research were as follows:

KEY FINDINGS OF THE RESEARCH

⌘ In terms of knowledge, understanding and technical skills for intensive care nursing, students who completed the online course were no different from students on the 'taught' course.

⌘ There is no evidence that students learn differently. However, the data indicated that e-learning, and supported distance learning, had a positive influence on the pilot students' learning and IT skills. This was especially so for time management and prioritising work.

⌘ Students, teachers and preceptors rated highly the virtual campus (ELEN) as a means of communication.

⌘ Release for study was 'tailored' to the needs of the student and the unit, and was adequate, and at the right time, for each student.

⌘ The preceptor's role with online students was little different from that with classroom-based students. However, the preceptors indicated that working with the online students had improved their awareness of the course content and individual student's progress.

⌘ Student and preceptor orientation programmes and accompanying support materials were effective.

⌘ Workload for teachers initially increased for the online cohort, but the teachers valued the opportunity and ability to work with students individually online.

As a result of the evaluation, some changes were made before rolling the online programme out more widely. First, the learning activities were reviewed and were reduced in number to minimise repetition. The activities were also structured around themes of the discussion groups. A second change was to include assessment of contribution to online discussion as part of the module-marking schedule. Some interesting comments emerged from the evaluative research:

> '... resulted in research-based practice and a logical and analytical approach to problems faced daily in an ICU.'
>
> (Preceptor)

'I think this course makes you learn more than a classroom course. You can spend a day in a classroom without learning anything, not listening. But on this course you have to gain your knowledge. There is no one else who does it for you.'

(Online student)

The above quote reflects the work of Biggs (1999) mentioned earlier in this chapter.

'... improved my awareness of the theory aspects of my work, challenged my existing knowledge, and also encouraged me to analyse my own and others' practice.'

(Online student)

Thames Valley University now uses Blackboard 5.0 as its e-learning platform, and the Adult Intensive Care Course has been converted to Blackboard.

The potential for this way of learning

Our experiences in delivering this uniprofessional online programme have enabled us to develop knowledge, skills and confidence in delivering an online clinical programme. We are exploring the potential for converting it to a multiprofessional online course for all healthcare professionals working in adult intensive care settings, to enhance interprofessional practice. Blackboard 5.0 makes it easy to add, delete and modify electronic learning materials and learning activities. The discussion groups could function as online multiprofessional learning sets, working through 'real-world' problems together. The social constructivist nature of the design of this online programme would facilitate multiprofessional learning with minimal modification.

A second potential for the future is the development of online programmes to prepare all healthcare clinical supervisors and preceptors. Many healthcare professions require their clinical supervisors and preceptors to undergo preceptor training. These preceptorship skills, however, are generic across all healthcare professional groups. Currently, clinical staff are required to be released from the workplace to undertake programmes of preparation to become clinical preceptors/supervisors. Our experience with this programme has led to the realisation that online multiprofessional clinical supervisor/preceptorship training is the way forward, obviating the need for clinical staff to be released from their place of work.

Conclusions

This chapter has presented social constructivist theory as underpinning multiprofessional and online learning, and illustrated this by two case studies of course design and delivery. Many institutions are engaged in multiprofessional, interprofessional and online course delivery, yet there is little in the published literature to indicate how different approaches to learning might influence the design, approach to, and delivery of the curriculum.

It is our belief that a thorough understanding of classic and social constructivist theories enables appropriate decisions to be made about the design and delivery of interprofessional and online courses, ensuring that learning is the focus. Additionally, we highlight the value of undertaking evaluative research into such initiatives, and how evaluative research leads to evidence-based curriculum development.

References

Biggs JB (1999) *Teaching for Quality Learning at University*. Society for Research in Higher Education and Open University Press, Buckingham

Black JB, McClintock RO (1995) An interpretation construction approach to curriculum design. http://www.ilt.columbia.edu/ilt/papers/ICON.html Columbia University, New York, accessed Feb 2002

Boulton D, Hammersley M (1996) Analysis of unstructured data. In: Sapsford R, Lupp, V (Eds). *Data Collection and Analysis*. Sage, London

Brown JS, Collins A, Duguid P (1998) Situated cognition and the culture of learning. http://www.ilt.columbia.edu/ilt/papers/John.Brown.html Columbia University, New York, accessed Feb 2002

Clarke A (2001) *Learning Organisations: What they are and how to become one*. National Institute of Adult Continuing Education (England & Wales), Leicester

Lave J, Wenger E (1991) *Situated Learning: Legitimate peripheral participation*. Cambridge University Press, Cambridge

Malhotra Y (1996) *Organisational Learning and Learning Organizations: An overview*. http://www.brint.com/papers/orglrng.htm, accessed Feb 2002

Mohr N, Dichter A (2001) Building a learning organisation. *Phi Delta Kappan* **82**(10): 744–50

Pawson R, Tilley N (1997) *Realistic Evaluation*. Sage, London

Penn-Handwerker W (2001) *Quick Ethnography*. Alta Mira Press, Walnut Creek, California

Piaget J (1972) *Insights and Illusions of Philosophy*. Routledge & Kegan Paul, New York

Prestine N A (1993) Extending the essential schools metaphor: principal as enabler. *Journal of School Leadership* **3**(4): 356–79

Renshaw P (1995) Excellence in teaching and learning. In: Lingard B, Rizva F (Eds). *External Environmental Scan*. Department of Education, Queensland, Australia

Senge PM (1990) *The Fifth Discipline*. Doubleday, New York

Senge PM, Kleiner A, Roberts C, Ross R B, Roth G, Smith BJ (1994) *The Fifth Discipline Fieldbook*. Nicholas Brealey, London

Senge PM, Kleiner A, Roberts C, Ross R B, Royh G, Smith BJ (1999) *The Dance of Change*. Nicholas Brealey, London

Senge PM (2002) Creating Quality Communities. http://www.sol-ne.org/res/Kr/qualcom.html. Society of Organizational Learning, *This is a 'virtual' site, web-based, and therefore has no specific location. Checked, and it is still 'live'.*

Strauss A, Corbin J (1990) *Basis of Qualitative Research: Grounded theory procedures and techniques*. Sage, Newbury Park, California

Tosey P (1999) The peer learning community: a contextual design for learning? *Management Decisions* **37**(5): 403–10

United Kingdom Central Council for Nursing, Midwifery and Health Visiting (UKCC) (1999) *Fitness for Practice (The Peach Report)*. UKCC, London

Vygotsky LS (1978) *Mind and Society: The development of higher psychological processes*. Harvard University, Cambridge, Massachusetts

Wenger E (1998) *Communities of Practice: Learning, meaning, and identity*. Cambridge University Press, Cambridge

13

Enabling interprofessional education: the potential of e-learning

Mike Farrell

The modernisation of the NHS has become a major policy objective, with efforts prioritised on ensuring delivery of a health service that is firmly based on the needs of patients (Department of Health [DoH], 2000). If this aspiration is to be realised, significant changes in the education of health professionals are required. Interprofessional education (IPE) has an important contribution to make in enabling health professionals to support the development of a modernised health service (Finch, 2000) and there is now significant interest in developing curricula with a strong interprofessional component.

If IPE is to be effectively realised, new approaches to its delivery are also required. There is now a move to explore how new learning technologies, particularly e-learning, can be used in the education of health professionals. The DoH (1998, 2001) has urged the increased and more effective use of e-learning.

This chapter will consider how e-learning approaches might be used to support the delivery of IPE, identifying key factors that have influenced a growth in interest and use of e-learning. The concept of e-learning will be reviewed, and specific learning conditions to promote a beneficial learning experience will be outlined.

The growth of e-learning

The benefits of e-learning are now significant. E-learning is strategically driven at regional, national and international levels, as evidenced by its inclusion as a key education and economic policy imperative (Commission of the European Union, 2001a; Department for Education and Skills [DfES], 2003). It is suggested that providers and funders of education must review their approaches and inform new developments in educational policy, investment priorities and learning infrastructure (Parrish and Parrish, 2000). Key drivers for the interest and growth in the use of e-learning include:

✿ *Developments in technology*: Technological developments enable the flexible integration and configuration of vast amounts of information from a diverse range of sources. Coupled with the ability to present such information using a variety of multimedia, e-learning can be packaged in a way that meets individual learning needs and styles (Wagner, 2000; Martinez, 2002;

Oakes, 2002). The use of intelligent monitoring–feedback technologies, such as Learning Management Systems (LMS) offers tremendous potential to personalise and track learner experiences, and monitor individual development.

✣ ***Developments in broadband technologies:*** These have substantial potential to enhance the delivery of internet services, particularly with regard to improved capacity and data-handling capabilities. Technological developments will significantly improve e-learning experiences by providing richer and more interactive e-learning environments.

✣ ***The rise of the knowledge-based economy:*** The realisation that the application of knowledge in the right way, at the right time, and by the right person offers economic advantage has been a main driver in growth of the knowledge-based economy (Morgan Keegan, 2000). Nowhere is this knowledge application more advantageous than in healthcare systems, where it helps to ensure effective and safe patient care. The use of e-learning as a platform for education and dissemination of knowledge is critical to the success of a knowledge-based economy (Commission of the European Communities, 2001b; Organisation for Economic Co-operation and Development [OECD], 2001).

✣ ***Limitations in available educational infrastructure:*** One of the key aims of current UK government policy is to increase the number of students entering higher education (DfES, 2003). While this aspiration is welcomed, there are concerns that the physical limitations in the current higher education infrastructure might prove a barrier. The use of e-learning is one way in which this limitation might be overcome. Crucially, it also extends educational opportunities, giving learners more choice about how and when they undertake their learning (DfES, 2003).

✣ ***The rise of corporate universities:*** The NHS University was created in 2003. This reflected an increasing interest in the development of the corporate university. Essentially, the purpose of such universities is to deliver a range of education and training programmes to the workforce of large corporations, which can be diverse both in training needs and geographical spread (Bjarnason *et al*, 2000). These organisations provide training and education explicitly linked to the achievement of clearly defined goals, with e-learning approaches as a main delivery channel.

What is e-learning?

Approach, format, content and benefits

E-learning is the facilitation of learning through the use of electronic technology. Although e-learning is a relatively recent innovation, already it can take different forms, with a variety of terms being used to describe it, including e-education, online learning and web-based training (Roffe, 2002). It has evolved from traditional distance learning education (Farrell, 2001).

When used effectively, e-learning can generate significant benefits for learners, educators and organisations. However, e-learning can have considerable disadvantages and must be critically evaluated to justify its appropriateness. *Table 13.1* lists some of the reported advantages and disadvantages of e-learning.
E-learning content can be offered in different formats and delivered via the Internet, Intranet, CD-ROM and DVD. Given the global adoption of the Internet, it is likely to become the main mode of delivery of e-learning. In the future, however, digital television is like ly to be a more important portal for e-learning than a personal computer.

Learning content can be offered using a variety of audiovisual media software and devices such as video and flash animation, with a potential for highly visual and engaging educational experiences. E-learning offers flexibility in the delivery of education: this can be immediate, delivered by an 'online' educator, or prepackaged learning material that learners can access at any time, and at a duration that is most convenient for them. Other forms of electronic communication such as e-mail and online discussion groups can be used to support and enhance the e-learning experience. These mechanisms enable interaction between learners and their peers, learners and educators, with the further potential to interact with a range of 'virtual communities'.

Applications of e-learning

E-learning has been most widely applied in the delivery of information technology (IT) skills training. It has also become popular in the support of management skills such as leadership and team building. The interest and growth in e-learning in the business sector is largely due to the economics of cost reduction in the provision of education and training.

In higher education, e-learning approaches deliver a range of academic courses online. In Australia, a national survey of online university courses has demonstrated that this approach is offered within a range of subject areas (Alexander, 2001). The adoption of e-learning by academic institutions in the UK reflects enterprise opportunities, but in many cases is simply supplementary to existing provision.

Table 13.1: Advantages and disadvantages of e-learning

Advantages	Available anytime/anywhere
	Accommodates different learning styles
	Allows self-paced learning
	Offers 'just-in-time' training
	Usability
	Can build self-confidence in the use of ICT technologies
	Encourages student's responsibility for learning
	Highly flexible/interactive possibility
	Scalability to workforce
	Rapid and total ability to update content of programmes
	Rapid distribution of education material/content to learning network
	Cost reduction
	Benefits for more efficient use of other learning resources, e.g. trainers, facilities
	Can be used to monitor the performance development of the individual/workforce
Disadvantages	Need for electronic access
	Needs IT knowledge and skills
	Lack of operability between IT platforms
	Lack of face-to-face contact
	Requires high learner motivation
	Potential user cost issues

E-learning and interprofessional education

IPE is characterised by the ability to foster collaborative learning opportunities between groups of health and social care professionals. The new learning technologies can support IPE. An example of this is the new interprofessional health curriculum being developed by the University of Southampton, which has utilised new learning technologies as a delivery channel http://www. commonlearning. net/project/index.htm. However, e-learning has not featured significantly in a number of important statements (Goosey and Barr, 2000; Barr, 2001) relating to IPE.

A number of factors can limit the opportunity for IPE within healthcare. Examples include:

- a workforce distributed across geographical distances
- a lack of expertise in IPE delivery
- pressure to meet clinical priorities.

Additionally, each learner may have individual reasons for finding face-to-face IPE a challenging learning situation. This could include:

- sensitivities about the issues being explored
- professional exposure
- disproportional mix of professional groups.

IPE delivered in electronic form can go some way to addressing structural and personal impediments to the learning process. E-learning offers a flexible and personal way of providing IPE that meets individual learning styles and needs, while retaining the interactive nature between professionals.

Healthcare education requires a high level of human interaction. It is possible that e-learning could reduce opportunities for human interaction and therefore be of limited benefit. However, with the integrated use of communication technologies such as synchronised video/audio conferences, discussion and bulletin boards, e-learning programmes can provide an alternative form of interactgiona nd communication.

Supporting communities of practice

E-learning approaches are frequently used to support the development of communities of practice – defined as a group of people who come together to share and learn from one another. By sharing knowledge, problems, experiences and best practice, group members broaden their knowledge and practice base (Kimble *et al*, 2001; Van Winkelen, 2003). While communities of practice can be created and located within small organisations, they can also, with the benefits of communication technologies, have a global membership. Thus communities of practice can benefit from a membership that reflects diverse social systems, cultures, values and experiences, which can enrich understanding and practice.

For some interprofessional programmes there could well be benefits in drawing on the theory of communities of practice to encourage ongoing interaction between learners within and beyond the completion of a formal education programme (Lave and Wenger, 1991). The use of an e-learning platform to deliver virtual tutor/learner led teaching sessions, or enable e-meetings to allow discussion and exchange of ideas can be a valuable mechanism in supporting a community of practice (Van Winkelen, 2003).

Interprofessional education (IPE) — a blended approach

In some situations, e-learning is inappropriate for meeting education or training needs. Careful assessment must ensure appropriateness of 'fit' between the required learning and the best way to achieve it. The integration of e-learning with other traditional methods is currently the subject of debate (Little, 2001; Mitchel, 2001; Voci and Young, 2001; Fraza, 2002). A 'blended approach' combines different traditional delivery methods, including didactic approaches, with electronic means of delivery.

A range of factors will determine the configuration of delivery methods. Such factors include desired learning outcomes, needs of learners, logistical issues such as number, profile and distribution of learners, and the availability of human and technological resources.

A blended approach promotes consolidation of learning by allowing students to re-engage with content following initial delivery by teaching staff. Conversely, a blended approach can be used to provide baseline knowledge and skills before a more structured learning event, making effective use of both educator and student time. This is particularly important, given that much IPE is provided at post-qualification level where learners might have to be released from service commitments in order to attend a learning event. Employers and learners need to feel confident that any scheduled learning time is used to maximum benefit. *Figure 13.1* gives some examples of how a blended approach might be used to deliver some common interprofessional learning activities.

Ensuring an effective e-learning experience

Educators will need to ensure that appropriate conditions are created if e-learning is to be used as an effective method to support the delivery of IPE. The intended learning outcomes must be the trigger for the design and content of any e-learning solution (Fry, 2001; Li Shen, 2002; Moyer, 2002). There has been a tendency for educators to simply reformat existing paper-based learning materials into an electronic format. While some materials can be used effectively, the reformat of others could impair the e-learning experience by being no more than e-reading (Honey, 2001). It is critical that the design of e-learning programme is based upon the learners' needs (Kruper, 2002).

UNDERTAKING BASIC CLINICAL OBSERVATIONS

Pulse, blood pressure, respiration & temperature recording

Target audience: Students of all health professions

Introduction to the basic principles of patient assessment
❖ E-learning format
❖ Electronic pre-assessment of the required competencies to be achieved

Undertaking clinical observations

❖ Electronic step-by-step simulation of specific procedures
❖ Work station hands-on experience in clinical skills lab, facilitated by clinical instructors
❖ One-to-one supervision in clinical area by clinical mentors

Maintaining clinical competency

❖ Periodic electronic assessment
❖ Drop-in update clinical skill sessions
❖ Evidence base update alert sent via email
❖ Electronic record of competence achieved integrated into electronic portfolio of development

EFFECTIVE MULTIPROFESSIONAL TEAM-WORKING

Target audience: Members of the multiprofessional team/students of all health professions

Introduction to the principles of effective interprofessional team-working

❖ Electronic asynchronous presentation of principles of effective team-working
❖ Multimedia presentation of key roles and function of different members of the healthcare team (video/audio/text/diagrams)
❖ Electronic case study presentations of interprofessional team-working (video/audio vignettes)
❖ Electronic assessment of knowledge of principles of multiprofessional team-working

Multiprofessional team-working – understanding values/attitudes/motives

Facilitator-led, face-to-face structured experiential session:
❖ Value/attitudes exploration
❖ Group discussion
❖ Role play

Sustaining awareness

❖ Electronic discussion group
❖ Provide electronic access to knowledge management resources

Figure 13.1: Examples of the application of e-learning to support interprofessional learning

Support for learners from educators will be a key factor in enabling them to benefit from the use of any e-learning approach. While this support can be provided using 'virtual' or face-to-face methods, it will be important to ensure that the learner can access that support at a time of need. If this is not available, the student may experience a loss of confidence, which could impact upon the quality of his or her learning experience. Engaging and providing support for learners using e-learning methods has implications for educators, who will need to develop new skills appropriate to the methods and technology employed (Commission of the European Communities, 2001c). Lack of expertise could lead to antipathy towards the use of this learning approach (Ryan, 2001). Some organisations have developed specific standards to identify the competencies that will be required by educators and trainers seeking to support learners in the use of e-learning-based programmes (for an example, access http://www.iitt. org.uk/public/standards/etutorcomp.asp).

The need for e-learning standards

There is a consensus that quality is crucial to the success of e-learning (Wagner, 2000; Farrell, 2001; E-learning Consortium, 2002). Significant attempts are now being made by the academic community and the e-learning industry to develop a standards framework to inform the design, access, interoperability, and indexing of e-learning programmes and services. For example, the Centre for Educational Technology Interoperability Standards (http://www.cetis.ac.uk) provides an extensive range of resources. Educators seeking to design and deliver programmes that include IPE with an e-learning format or component will need to be familiar with the appropriate standards for their subject area.

A successful e-learning experience is dependent upon access to a robust, well-maintained stable technology infrastructure (Anderson and Jackson, 2000; Wagner, 2000; Alexander, 2001; Henry, 2001). Technical problems and limitations can be frustrating for learners and may adversely affect their learning experience (Ryan, 2001).

As part of the delivery of any programme, educators will need to assess the availability of access to software and hardware devices (including level of specification), and any necessary technical support, to learners. They will need to ensure that programmes can be delivered across an agreed minimum technological specification.

The importance of reusable learning objects

Developing high-quality learning content for delivery using e-learning methods can be particularly expensive and lengthy. There is now considerable interest in developing 'learning objects' (Shaw and Sniderman, 2002; Polsani, 2003). These are best described as a breakdown of learning content into discrete re-usable elements, shared across courses and organisations (Shaw and Sniderman, 2002). Learning objects can be considered the building blocks of an electronic programme and can take many forms, including web pages, PDF documents, and database applications (Oliver, 2001). The configuration of the individual learning objects, which have been specifically designed to achieve a planned learning outcome, will be a critical element in ensuring an effective learning experience.

Since collaboration is the core principle of IPE, it should be reflected in the design of materials. However, such collaboration requires leadership, openness and a commitment to sharing by academic staff. The potential of what can be achieved is illustrated by current collaborative developments in the UK (see Universities' Collaboration in eLearning (UCEL) at http://www.ucel.ac.uk or The Students On-Line in Nursing Integrated Curricula (SONIC) project at http://www.uclan.ac.uk/facs/health/nursing/sonic/).

Conclusion

Developments in e-learning offer significant potential as a valuable approach to support the education of health professionals, including the delivery of IPE. This chapter has outlined key aspects of e-learning and suggested ways in which this method might be applied to support the delivery of IPE.

Author's note

This chapter is based upon Farrell M (2002) *E-Learning and the Local Health NHS Workforce: Drivers, essential conditions, challenges and opportunities.* Cumbria and Lancashire Workforce Development Confederation.

References

Alexander S (2001) E-learning developments and experiences. *Education and Training* **43**(4/5): 240–8

Anderson M, Jackson D (2000) Computer systems for distributed and distance learning. *Journal of Computer Assisted Learning* **16**: 213-28

Barr H (2001) *Interprofessional Education Today, Yesterday and Tomorrow– A review* @ www.health.ltsn.ac.uk/miniprojects/HughBarrFinal.htm Accessed 4 July 2003

Bjarnason S, Davies J, Farrington D *et al. The Business of Borderless Education: UK Perspectives. Summary Report.* THE VCP and Higher Education Funding Council for England @ www.universitiesuk.ac.uk/bookshop/downloads/BorderlessSummary.pdf Accessed 4 July 2003

Commission of the European Communities (2001a) *eLearning: Designing Tomorrow's Education.* Commission of the European Communities, Brussels

Commission of the European Communities (2001b) *eEurope 2002: European Youth into the Digital Age.* Commission of the European Communities, Brussels

Commission of the European Communities (2001c) *eEurope 2002: Impact and Priorities.* Commission of the European Communities, Brussels

Department for Education and Skills (DfES) (2003) *The Future of Higher Education. Department for Education and Skills.* The Stationery Office, London

Department of Health (1998) *Information for Health.* HMSO, London

Department of Health (2000) *The NHS Plan: A plan for investment. A plan for Reform.* HMSO, London

Department of Health (2001) *Working Together – Learning Together. A Framework for Lifelong Learning in the NHS.* HMSO, London

e-Learning Consortium (2002) *Making Sense of Learning Specifications & Standards: A Decision Maker's Guide to their Adoption.* The Masie Center @ www.masie.com/ standards/S3_Guide.pdf Accessed 4 July 2003

Farrell G (2001) *The Changing Faces of Virtual Education.* The Commonwealth of Learning @ www.col.org/virtualed/index2.htm accessed 4 July 2003

Finch J (2000) Interprofessional education and team-working: a view from education providers. *BMJ* **321**: 1138-40

Fraza V (2002) Training in the electronic classroom. *Industrial Distribution* **January** @ www.p21.com/press/id-electronic-classroom.html Accessed 4 July 2003

Fry K (2001) E-learning Markets and providers: some issues and prospects. *Education and Training* **43**(4/5): 233–9

Goosey D, Barr H (2002) *Selected Case Studies of Interprofessional Education.* Centre for the Advancement of Interprofessional Education @ http://www.caipe.org.uk/ documents/DOHcasestudies.pdf, *accessed 30th June 2003*

Henry P (2001) E-learning technology, content and services. *Education and Training* **43**(4): 249–55

Honey P (2001) E-learning: a performance appraisal and some suggestions for improvement. *The Learning Organisation* **8**(5): 200–2

Kimble C, Hildreth P, Wright P (2001) Communities of practice: going virtual. In: Malhotra Y (Ed). *Knowledge Management and Business Model Innovation*. Idea Group Publishing, Hershey, USA: 220–34

Kruper J (2002) Putting the learner front and center: using user-centred design principles to build better e-learning products. *The eLearning Developers' Journal* **March**: 8–11

Lave J, Wenger E (1991) *Situated Learning: Legitimate peripheral participation.* Cambridge University Press, Cambridge

Little B (2001) Achieving high performance through e-learning. *Education and Training* **33**(6): 203–7

McMahon J, Gardner J, Gray C, Mulhearn G (1999) Barriers towards computer usage: staff and students' perceptions. *Journal of Computer Assisted Learning* **15**: 302–11

Martinez M (2002) What is personalised learning? *The e-Learning Developers' Journal* **May** @ http://www.elearningguild.com/pbuild/linkbuilder. cfm?selection=fol.38 Accessed 23 June 2002

Mitchell L (2001) E-learning methods offer a personalized approach. *InfoWorld* @ http://archive.infoworld.com/articles/tc/xml/01/04/16/010416tcelearning.xml Accessed 4 July 2003

Morgan Keegan (2000) *eLearning: The Engine of the Knowledge Economy* @ suned. sun.com/US/images/executive_morgan.pdf Accessed 4 July 2003

Moyer LG (2002) Is digital learning effective in the workplace? *eLearn Magazine* @ http://elearnmag.org/subpage/sub_page.cfm?section=7&list_item=2&page=1 Accessed 4 July 2003

Oakes K (2002) *E-Learning. Training and Development* **56**(9): 57

Oliver R (2001) Learning objects: supporting flexible delivery of flexible learning. In: Kennedy G, Keppell M, McNaught C, Petrovic T (Eds). *Meeting at the Crossroads: Proceedings of ASCILITE 2001*. The University of Melbourne, Melbourne: 453-60

Parrish DM, Parrish AW (2000) *Developing a Distance Education Policy for 21st Century Learning*. Division of Government Public Affairs, American Council on Education, Washington

Polsani P (2003) Use and abuse of reusable learning objects. Journal of Digital Information V3 (4) From http://jodi.ecs.soton.ac.uk/Articles/v03/i04/Polsani Accessed 30 June 2003

Roffe I (2002) E-learning: engagement, enhancement and execution. *Quality Assurance in Education* **10**(1): 40–50

Ryan Y. The provision of learner support services online. In: Farrell G (2001) *The Changing Faces of Virtual Education*. The Commonwealth of Learning: 71-94. Available @ www.col.org/virtualed/index2.htm Accessed 23 June 2002

Shaw S, Sniderman S (2002) *Reusable Learning Objects: Critique and future directions*. Available @ http://www.aace.org/dl/files/ELEARN2002/paper_3009_ 3403.pdf Accessed 4 July 2003

Van Winkelen C (2003) *Inter-Organizational Communities of Practice*. Elearningeuropa.info available @ http://www.elearningeuropa.info/doc.php?id=14 83&lng=1&doclng=1 Accessed 4 July 2003

Voci E, Young K (2001) Blended learning working in a leadership development programme. *Industrial and Commercial Training* **33** (5): 157–60

Wagner ED. Emerging Technology Trends in e-Learning. *LineZine* **Fall** 2000 available @ http://www.linezine.com/2.1/features/ewette.htm Accessed 4 July 2003

Weller M (2000) Implementing a CMC tutor group for an existing distance education course. *Journal of Computer Assisted Learning* **16**: 178–83

Young K (2001) The effective deployment of e-learning. *Industrial and Commercial Training* **33** (1): 5–11

14

Evaluating interprofessional education

Hugh Barr

Like audit, monitoring, review, evaluation and research, interprofessional education (IPE) is a seemingly precise term accorded many meanings. Opting though it must for one overarching term, this chapter is nevertheless more concerned with purpose, process and outcomes than semantics. It summarises ways in which IPE has been evaluated, as reported in surveys and reviews, introduces questions framed by the UK Centre for the Advancement of Interprofessional Education (CAIPE, 2002) and takes into account benchmarking for undergraduate IPE in the UK. It ends with recommendations for good practice.

Findings from surveys and reviews

A UK survey of IPE initiatives undertaken in 1991 revealed that while nine-tenths had, according to respondents, been evaluated, only a quarter of these had been written up and still fewer published. Evaluation was most frequently based upon participants' satisfaction, although half reported that they took the opinions of other stakeholders into account. Half also said that they had employed before and after measures to record changes in participants' attitudes or perceptions, while others said they had observed the impact of learning on collaborative practice (Barr and Waterton, 1996).

The survey confirmed the experience of Barr and Shaw (1995) who had found only 19 published UK evaluations from an online library search and their knowledge of the field. Reports differed in the degree to which they exposed methodology to critical review. Some obliged readers to take research methods and data on trust. Others spelt out both, notably McMichael *et al* (1984), Gill and Ling (1994), Shaw (1994), Carpenter (1995a,b) and Carpenter and Hewstone (1996).

Evaluations took into account one or more of the following:

- programme planning, development and delivery
- learning process
- participants and their participation
- participant's satisfaction with the learning
- participants' assessment of their learning
- changes in participants' attitudes, perceptions and/or knowledge
- impact on participants' practice.

Data were collected by observation, questionnaire and sometimes interview. Most college-based courses limited attempts to measure outcomes to stated course objectives.

Five years later, the Interprofessional Education Joint Evaluation Team (JET) also selected nineteen evaluations to include in its UK literature review, from forty considered (Barr *et al*, 2000). (Of the nineteen, Barr and Shaw, 1995, had included four.) Teachers and trainers had conducted most of the evaluations themselves. These tended to be formative, concerned more with stakeholder satisfaction than meeting externally determined criteria. Methods again included questionnaires, interviews and observation, but there were also focus groups and analyses of students' essays.

Ten studies evaluated student satisfaction. Twelve reported changes in attitude towards colleagues and other professions. Fewer reported acquisition of knowledge, only seven reported changes in practice, and only two reported direct benefit to service users, in one case improved immunisation and cervical cytology rates (Thomas, 1994) and in the other improved diabetic control (Hutt, 1994).

This UK review was a spin-off from JET's main work, which comprises two systematic reviews of databases for evaluations of IPE worldwide.* The first has been completed (Zwarenstein *et al*, 1999, 2001) and the second is close to completion at the time of writing (see Freeth *et al*, 2002, for the most recent report).

Both were restricted to IPE where:

> *'Members (or students) of two or more professions associated with health or social care were engaged in learning with, from and about each other.'*
> (Zwarenstein *et al*, 1999)

The research question, however, differed. The first review asked simply:

> *'Does IPE work?'*
> (Zwarenstein *et al*, 2001)

The second asked:

> *'What kind of IPE works under what circumstances?'*
> (Freeth *et al*, 2002)

The first review was conducted under the auspices of the Cochrane Collaboration, subject to agreed criteria as follows. Evaluations had to comprise randomised controlled trials, controlled before and after studies, or interrupted time-series studies, and had to report outcomes demonstrating direct benefit to patients or clients. None were found that met both criteria.

The second review takes into account a wider range of research methodologies

---

*The Cochrane Group for the first review comprised Merrick Zwarenstein, Jo Atkins, Hugh Barr

than the Cochrane Review and a continuum of outcomes. By April 2002, 162 papers had been included from Medline (1968–2000), 179 from CINAHL (1982–2001) and three from the British Educational Index (BEI) (1964–2001) from more than 6000 abstracts checked. Allowing for the 124 papers appearing in both Medline and CINAHL, the total number of evaluations included in the review was 217 at that time, and was expected to rise as other databases were searched.

Of the 217 evaluations included, 184 (85%) had been published since 1990, and 128 (59%) since 1995, reflecting both the growth in IPE and its evaluation. More were based in hospitals (104; 48%) than in the community (87; 40%), the remainder being in both or unclear. Substantially more were post-qualifying (150; 69%) than pre-qualifying education (55; 25%), the remainder being mixed.

Most were from the USA (170; 78%), followed by the UK (26; 12%); the remainder were from Australia, Canada, Norway and Turkey. The relevance of US evaluations to UK education and practice is open to challenge, given their fundamental differences in education and healthcare systems, but the programmes described, research methods used and findings are sufficiently similar to those from the UK to encourage comparison.

The research designs employed were classified as shown in *Table 14.1*.

Positive outcomes reported were classified as shown in *Table 14.2*, using a modified version of the scale formulated by Kirkpatrick (1967).

Table 14.1: Classification of research designs employed (N = 217)

Research design	No. (%)	
Post-intervention, single time point	56	(26%)
Post-intervention, single time point, with control	6	(3%)
Post-intervention with follow-up	6	(3%)
During and after study	1	(<1%)
Before and after study	46	(21%)
Controlled before and after	8	(4%)
Before, during and after	6	(3%)
Before and after with follow-up	11	(5%)
Longitudinal	45	(21%)
Longitudinal with control group	2	(<1%)
Randomised controlled trial	1	(<1%)
Action research	1	(<1%)
Case study	1	(<1%)
Not given	27	(12%)

Table 14.2: Classification of positive outcomes (N = 217)		
Positive outcome	**No.**	**(%)**
Learners' reactions	96	(44%)
Modification of attitudes/perceptions	33	(15%)
Acquisition of knowledge/skills	78	(36%)
Change in individual behaviour	49	(22%)
Change organisation of practice	93	(42%)
Benefit to patients	47	(21%)

These outcomes were tabulated against characteristics of IPE, such as location, duration of the course, stage in participants' experience and structure included in the provisional typology floated by Barr (1996).

Analyses of the JET data found correlations between outcomes and duration and location of the course.

⌘ Comparison of positive outcomes with duration of the learning showed that short programmes (one day to two weeks) were more likely than long programmes (>2 weeks) to change practice and benefit patients (*Table 14.3*).

⌘ Comparison of positive outcomes with the location of the learning showed that work-based programmes were far more like to change practice and benefit patients directly (*Table 14.4*).

It must be borne in mind that university-based programmes rarely aim to do more than modify attitudes. Furthermore, measuring impact on practice is problematic, given that students come from or enter many different places of work.

A review by Cooper *et al* (2000, 2001) is broader and narrower than the JET review: broader in that inclusion criteria extended beyond evaluation, and narrower in that it focused upon undergraduate education. Like JET, Cooper and colleagues developed an alternative to the Cochrane protocol. They found wide variations in methodological rigour, including:

• selection bias — lack of controls
• attrition bias — lack of information on attrition rates
• detection bias — differences in the methods used to assess outcomes and selective reporting of results
• use of non-validated instruments to measure outcomes
• inadequate description of statistical analysis.

Table 14.3: Comparison of positive outcomes and duration of IPE

Positive outcome	Short programme (n=67)	Long programme (n=132)
Reactions	49 (73%)	41 (31%)
Attitudes	13 (19%)	15 (11%)
Knowledge	38 (57%)	33 (25%)
Individual behaviour	14 (21%)	29 (22%)
Organisational practice	13 (19%)	72 (55%)
Patient benefit	3 (4%)	39 (29%)

Table 14.4: Comparison of positive outcomes and location of IPE

Positive outcome	University (n=47)	Work (n=152)
Reactions	33 (70%)	46 (30%)
Attitudes	13 (28%)	14 (9%)
Knowledge	30 (64%)	37 (24%)
Individual behaviour	7 (15%)	41 (27%)
Organisational practice	4 (9%)	89 (59%)
Patient benefit	1 (2%)	44 (29%)

Unlike the systematic reviews conducted by JET, the majority of the studies reviewed by Cooper *et al* (2000; 2001) had been published in the UK and included more undergraduate IPE than is likely to be found in other countries. Of 141 studies found, thirty were deemed to be sufficiently rigorous to include in the review, of which sixteen were classified as evaluations and fourteen as research studies. Of these fourteen, eleven used quantitative design and three qualitative design. Attention focused primarily on the measurement of process variables to ascertain whether the intervention was successfully applied and was operating in the expected direction. Questionnaires were the most common method, but only 35% of studies used validated instruments. New instruments were designed without considering reliability and validity.

Systematic reviews such as these are an expeditious, economic and effective way to locate evaluations that satisfy defined criteria. They are the best available means to establish what has been evaluated, how and by whom. Their consistency and transparency does much to reduce reviewer bias, to expose process to critical appraisal and to facilitate replication and updating.

But bias is not wholly eliminated. There is the time lag between completion of a programme, publication of its evaluation, entry in one or more databases and pick-up by a systematic review; more recent evaluations are missed. There is bias in the databases that reviewers choose to search and in the languages (invariably English) that databases and reviews cover. There is bias, too, in favour of 'success stories' in evaluations written up, submitted for publication and accepted by journals.

The quality of evaluations reported may therefore be atypical — the tip of the proverbial iceberg — with less rigorous and less positive evaluations beneath the surface. The fact that the quality of evaluations reported is uneven and reportage often incomplete does little to inspire confidence in the general standard of evaluation of interprofessional education.

Some critical questions

Evaluation of IPE draws upon methods employed in mainstream education. It must, however, take into account the distinguishing characteristics of IPE. The Centre for the Advancement of Interprofessional Education has therefore framed the following questions, which it invites individuals and organisations evaluating IPE to take into account (CAIPE, 2002).

Do the stated objectives claim to promote collaborative practice?
Noting that collaborative learning between professions can prepare for collaborative practice between agencies and with communities, service users and their carers, as well as between professions.

How are those claims substantiated?
Establishing whether content and learning methods can deliver the objectives that work towards collaborative practice.

Does the collaboration contribute to improving the quality of care?
Recognising that collaboration is only a means towards improvement in services, provision of care and patient benefit.

Are the objectives compatible?
Bearing in mind that promoting collaboration may be one of many objectives with different implications for structure, content and learning methods.

How is IPE built into the programme?
Ensuring that IPE is woven coherently into structure, content and learning methods throughout.

Is the programme informed by a theoretical rationale?
Introducing theoretical perspectives to inform programme design, teaching and learning about collaborative practice.

Is the programme evidence based?
Basing teaching and learning on evidence from research, including outcomes from systematic reviews of IPE and practice.

Is the programme informed by interprofessional values?
Helping to secure the value base for IPE and practice, and identifying common values across professions while also exploring differences between them.

Does comparative learning complement common learning?
Enabling participating professions to learn from and about each other to inform intelligent collaboration based on appreciation of each profession's distinctive contribution to practice.

Are learning methods interactive?
Employing a repertoire of interactive methods that engage participants in such exchange through joint assignments designed to facilitate comparative learning.

Is small group learning included?
Investing in small groups that optimise interactive learning, suitably accommodated with generous staff:student ratios.

Will numbers from each profession be balanced?
Recruiting, so far as is practicable, comparable numbers from each of the participating professions, introducing quotas if necessary.

Are all the professions represented in planning and teaching?
Involving teachers or trainers from all the participating professions in programme planning, delivery and evaluation.

Are service users and carers involved?
Involving service users and carers in programme design, teaching, assessment and evaluation, and as co-participants, to emphasise learning for user-centred service.

Will interprofessional learning be assessed and count towards qualification?
Adding to the value of interprofessional learning, in the eyes of participants, teachers, employers and others, by including it in assessment for awards.

Will the programme be evaluated?
Ensuring that all IPE is subject to audit or review and subjecting programmes to more systematic evaluation.

Will findings be disseminated?
Sharing lessons learned with comparable programmes in other institutions through conference presentations, reports and journal articles.

Benchmarking

Particular requirements apply to for the review of undergraduate IPE in the UK made by the Quality Assurance Agency (QAA) for Higher Education on behalf of the Department of Health and other government departments. These comprise benchmark statements for nursing and each of the allied health professions, formulated in consultation with representatives of each of those professions. Common statements have been agreed for common learning (QAA, 2001).

CAIPE welcomed the balance struck between statements specific to each and common to all these professions, especially the inclusion of statements about collaboration. It questioned, however, whether these were sufficient, without further work, to ensure that newly qualified workers would be ready for collaborative practice (Barr, 2002).

Evaluation in future

IPE takes many forms, calling for different approaches to evaluation, making different claims on resources. The evaluative design must be sensitive to the distinctive characteristics of each programme. Generalisation is hazardous and guidelines are premature. There is as much room for imagination and innovation in the evaluation of IPE as as there is in its design and delivery.

Some programmes merit more rigorous evaluation than others, for example, those that break new ground in the needs they address, the learning methods they employ or the professions they include. But they all require some evaluation.

Many evaluations are formative, designed to help teachers and students determine whether the programme has fulfilled its stated objectives, to assess the effectiveness of the methods employed, and to inform decisions about improvements for the benefit of future intakes. Methods such as questionnaires, focus groups and interviews may be used in much the same ways as for professional education, but introducing questions specific to interprofessional learning and the programme.

Useful though such evaluation may be, it does not suffice where the programme is subject to validation or review in accordance with externally determined criteria, whether external to the programme by the parent institution, or to the institution by, or on behalf of, the funding body. These evaluations have a formative element, but are essentially summative, working to a predetermined standard and judging one programme against others.

Each validating and funding body lays down its own requirements, which are designed primarily for professional, not interprofessional, education. The QAA benchmarking standards are a major step towards making that transition, having implications for education beyond undergraduate IPE. The questions framed by CAIPE focus on qualities that should characterise IPE, and which need to be taken into account in any evaluation. Both can be used mindlessly and mechanistically as no more than checklists. Value is added when they are woven into approaches to evaluation, such as those reported in this chapter.

Most IPE is likely to be evaluated in accordance with external criteria, now that it has entered the mainstream of professional education. Some programmes will merit more sustained, more searching, and more rigorous evaluation to extend the evidence base for IPE. It is here that the following principles apply especially.

⌘ Begin at the beginning

Evaluation must not be an afterthought. It should be built into plans for the programme from the outset, and be included in the budget. Without this, preparation may be hasty, resources inadequate, consultation poor, and cooperation half-hearted. Initial intakes may be omitted, or only picked up towards the end, and the opportunity to evaluate the planning stages missed.

⌘ Match objectives

Objectives for the evaluation should be based upon objectives for the programme — no more and no less — and be concerned as much with the means by which they are achieved as with whether they are achieved.

⌘ Evaluate process and outcomes

Account should therefore be taken of both process and outcomes. Too many evaluations set out to measure changes in attitude, perception or knowledge, without even describing the learning experience, still less evaluating it.

⌘ Choose your methods

Different professions may prefer different research methods. Scientifically based professions, such as medicine, may prefer quantitative methods using experimental designs and treating randomised controlled trials (RCTs) as the gold standard. Nursing, social work and education may prefer qualitative methods. Time needs to be set aside to debate the relative merits of different methods as applied to education in general, and professional education and IPE in particular.

RCTs are essential for clinical trials designed to determine the safety and effects of drugs and medical interventions, but qualitative methods find more favour for evaluating education.

Given that only two RCTs evaluating IPE have been reported (Freeth *et al*, 2002), there is a persuasive case for putting them to the test, although the ethical, logistical and practical obstacles are formidable, and the dividends, in isolation from other research methods, unclear. Moreover, RCTs, if and when applied to IPE, will need to be performed by experienced researchers.

A well-planned evaluation will probably use two or more research methods — mainly qualitative to evaluate process, and qualitative and quantitative to evaluate outcomes.

⌘ Include before and after measures

Feedback after the programme may assess student satisfaction and inform future change, but it is meaningless to measure learning from the programme. This requires before and after measures, consistently designed and applied, keeping attrition to a minimum. Longer programmes may well introduce measures at intervening points, for example, at the end of each module.

⌘ Follow-up

One better, the evaluation may follow up students, say six or twelve months later, inviting them to comment, with benefit of hindsight, on their learning, and to report any ways in which they have sought to apply it in their work. Verification of the latter may be sought from line managers and service users.

Follow-up moves towards evaluating the impact of the programme upon practice, but the findings must be treated with extreme caution, given that so many variables may intervene, and the difficulties in tracing former students and verifying what they say.

⌘ Build in controls

Experimental design, such as RCTs, may be the exception. Quasi-experimental design is more realistic, albeit uncommon, in evaluating IPE. Matched control groups can be introduced reasonably easily.

⌘ Use validated instruments

Few, if any, instruments have been designed and tested for express use in IPE, although some have been 'borrowed'. There is a pressing need to discuss and determine what kinds of instruments are needed, and then to commission work to design, test and validate them.

⌘ **Replicate**

While there may be distinctive features of a programme to be evaluated in a distinctive way, difference for difference's sake is to be avoided. Inexperienced researchers would be better advised to replicate well-tried methods. Reports of evaluations should pay sufficient attention to research methods to enable others to replicate them. This is far from so at present.

⌘ **Involve all possible parties**

IPE has many stakeholders, for example, students, teachers, managers, and not least service users. The more perspectives taken into account, the more rounded and persuasive may be the findings.

⌘ **Beware of bias**

Teachers conduct most evaluations of IPE themselves. These benefit from their intimate experience of their programmes, but are liable to bias. One way to reduce this risk is to retain a researcher experienced in this field as a consultant, to be called upon at critical stages in the process.

⌘ **Be realistic**

Above all, be realistic. Nothing serves IPE worse than ill-founded and exaggerated claims. The more ambitious the evaluation envisaged, the stronger the case for bringing in external researchers. Resource implications will, however, dictate that their services are called upon selectively for the most innovative programmes.

Conclusion

Those who assert that there is no evidence for the effectiveness of IPE are either behind the times or unwilling to accept the validity of research methods other than those with which they are familiar in clinical trials.

The evidence base is painstakingly being secured, but evaluations are widely scattered in time and place, and uneven in rigour. The best are, however, exemplary, providing pointers for future evaluations of IPE.

Additional evaluations are still being found as further databases are searched, but with diminishing returns. Many have already been reported in other databases. Enough is now known to define the baseline for future evaluations, the questions to be framed, the studies to be replicated, the methods to be employed, the instruments to be adopted, adapted or designed from scratch, and the pitfalls to be avoided.

References

Barr H (1966) Ends and means in IPE: towards a typology. *Education for Health* **9** (3): 341–52

Barr H (2002) CAIPE consulted on new benchmarks for training. *CAIPE Bulletin* **21**: 4

Barr H, Shaw I (1995) *Shared Learning: Selected examples from the literature.* CAIPE, London

Barr H, Waterton S (1996) *Interprofessional Education in Health and Social Care: Report of a CAIPE survey.* CAIPE, London

Barr H, Freeth D, Hammick M, Koppel I, Reeves S (2000) *Evaluations of Interprofessional Education: A United Kingdom review for health and social care.* CAIPE and the British Educational Research Association, London

CAIPE (2002) *Assuring the Quality of Interprofessional Education for Health and Social Care.* CAIPE, London

Carpenter J (1995a) Doctors and nurses: stereotypes and stereotype change in interprofessional education. *J Interprof Care* **9**: 151–62

Carpenter J (1995b) Interprofessional education for medical and nursing students: evaluation of a programme. *Med Educ* **29**: 256–72

Carpenter J, Hewstone M (1996) Shared learning for doctors and social workers: evaluation of a programme. *British Journal of Social Work* **26**: 239–57

Cooper H, Carlisle C, Gibbs T, Watkins C (2000) Using qualitative methods for conducting a systematic review. *Nurse Res* **8**(1): 28–38

Cooper H, Carlisle C, Gibbs T, Watkins C (2001) Developing an evidence base for interdisciplinary learning: a systematic review. *J Adv Nurs* **35**(2): 289–37

Freeth D, Hammick M, Koppel I, Reeves S, Barr H (2002) *A Critical Review of Evaluations of Interprofessional Education.* The Learning and Teaching Support Network for Health Sciences and Practice, London

Gill J, Ling J (1994) Interprofessional shared learning: a curriculum for collaboration. In: Soothill K, L Mackay L, Webb C (Eds). *Interprofessional Relations in Healthcare.* Edward Arnold, London: 172–93

Hutt M (1994) *Continuing Medical Education in Essex: Final report.* Anglia Polytechnic University, Chelmsford

Kirkpatrick DL (1967) Evaluation of training. In: Craig R, Bittel L (Eds). *Training and Development Handbook.* McGraw Hill, New York: 131–67

McMichael P, Irvine R, Gilloran A (1984) *Pathways to the Professions: Research report.* Moray House College of Education, Edinburgh

QAA (2001) *Benchmarking Academic and Practitioner Standards in Healthcare Subjects.* Quality Assurance Agency for Higher Education, Bristol

Shaw I (1994) *Evaluating Interprofessional Training*. Avebury, Aldershot

Thomas P (1994) *The Liverpool Primary Healthcare Facilitation Project 1989–1994*. The Liverpool Family Health Service Authority, Liverpool

Zwarenstein M, Atkins J, Barr H, Hammick M, Koppel I, Reeves S (1999) A systematic review of interprofessional education. *J Interprof Care* **13**(4): 417-24

Zwarenstein M, Reeves S, Barr H, Hammick M, Koppel I, Atkins J (2001) *Interprofessional Education: Effects on professional practice and health*. The Cochrane Collaboration, Oxford

Acknowledgements

I am indebted to fellow members of the Interprofessional Education Joint Evaluation Team — Dr Della Freeth, Dr Marilyn Hammick, Dr Ivan Koppel and Scott Reeves — for their comments on this chapter in draft and for allowing me to draw upon their wealth of experience.

Index